Fungal Infections Complicating COVID-19

Fungal Infections Complicating COVID-19

Editors

Martin Hoenigl
Alida Fe Talento

MDPI • Basel • Beijing • Wuhan • Barcelona • Belgrade • Manchester • Tokyo • Cluj • Tianjin

Editors
Martin Hoenigl
University of California
San Diego
USA

Alida Fe Talento
Royal College of Surgeons
Ireland

Editorial Office
MDPI
St. Alban-Anlage 66
4052 Basel, Switzerland

This is a reprint of articles from the Special Issue published online in the open access journal *Journal of Fungi* (ISSN 2309-608X) (available at: https://www.mdpi.com/journal/jof/special_issues/fungal_COVID-19).

For citation purposes, cite each article independently as indicated on the article page online and as indicated below:

LastName, A.A.; LastName, B.B.; LastName, C.C. Article Title. *Journal Name* **Year**, *Volume Number*, Page Range.

ISBN 978-3-0365-0554-1 (Hbk)
ISBN 978-3-0365-0555-8 (PDF)

Contents

About the Editors . . . . **vii**

Alida Fe Talento and Martin Hoenigl
Fungal Infections Complicating COVID-19: With the Rain Comes the Spores
Reprinted from: *J. Fungi* **2020**, *6*, 279, doi:10.3390/jof6040279 . . . . **1**

Amir Arastehfar, Agostinho Carvalho, Frank L. van de Veerdonk, Jeffrey D. Jenks, Philipp Koehler, Robert Krause, Oliver A. Cornely, David S. Perlin, Cornelia Lass-Flörl and Martin Hoenigl
COVID-19 Associated Pulmonary Aspergillosis (CAPA)—From Immunology to Treatment
Reprinted from: *J. Fungi* **2020**, *6*, 91, doi:10.3390/jof6020091 . . . . **3**

Jean-Pierre Gangneux, Florian Reizine, Hélène Guegan, Kieran Pinceaux, Pierre Le Balch, Emilie Prat, Romain Pelletier, Sorya Belaz, Mathieu Le Souhaitier, Yves Le Tulzo, Philippe Seguin, Mathieu Lederlin, Jean-Marc Tadié and Florence Robert-Gangneux
Is the COVID-19 Pandemic a Good Time to Include *Aspergillus* Molecular Detection to Categorize Aspergillosis in ICU Patients? A Monocentric Experience
Reprinted from: *J. Fungi* **2020**, *6*, 105, doi:10.3390/jof6030105 . . . . **21**

Aia Mohamed, Thomas R. Rogers and Alida Fe Talento
COVID-19 Associated Invasive Pulmonary Aspergillosis: Diagnostic and Therapeutic Challenges
Reprinted from: *J. Fungi* **2020**, *6*, 115, doi:10.3390/jof6030115 . . . . **33**

Eelco F. J. Meijer, Anton S. M. Dofferhoff, Oscar Hoiting, Jochem B. Buil and Jacques F. Meis
Azole-Resistant COVID-19-Associated Pulmonary Aspergillosis in an Immunocompetent Host: A Case Report
Reprinted from: *J. Fungi* **2020**, *6*, 79, doi:10.3390/jof6020079 . . . . **47**

Amir Arastehfar, Agostinho Carvalho, M. Hong Nguyen, Mohammad Taghi Hedayati, Mihai G. Netea, David S. Perlin and Martin Hoenigl
COVID-19-Associated Candidiasis (CAC): An Underestimated Complication in the Absence of Immunological Predispositions?
Reprinted from: *J. Fungi* **2020**, *6*, 211, doi:10.3390/jof6040211 . . . . **55**

Brunella Posteraro, Riccardo Torelli, Antonietta Vella, Paolo Maria Leone, Giulia De Angelis, Elena De Carolis, Giulio Ventura, Maurizio Sanguinetti and Massimo Fantoni
Pan-Echinocandin-Resistant *Candida glabrata* Bloodstream Infection Complicating COVID-19: A Fatal Case Report
Reprinted from: *J. Fungi* **2020**, *6*, 163, doi:10.3390/jof6030163 . . . . **69**

Ioannis Ventoulis, Theopisti Sarmourli, Pinelopi Amoiridou, Paraskevi Mantzana, Maria Exindari, Georgia Gioula and Timoleon-Achilleas Vyzantiadis
Bloodstream Infection by *Saccharomyces cerevisiae* in Two COVID-19 Patients after Receiving Supplementation of *Saccharomyces* in the ICU
Reprinted from: *J. Fungi* **2020**, *6*, 98, doi:10.3390/jof6030098 . . . . **81**

About the Editors

Martin Hoenigl M.D., Ass. Prof., FECMM, holds an appointment as Assistant Professor at the Division of Infectious Diseases of the University of California, San Diego (UCSD). He obtained his venia docendi in internal medicine in 2012 and is the author of over 200 PubMed-listed publications in the field of infectious diseases, the majority in leading authorship (i.e., first or last author; ORCiD: 0000-0002-1653-2824). His research is focused on clinical mycology, with a particular focus on diagnosis and lately COVID-associated aspergillosis. He serves as the current president of the European Confederation of Medical Mycology (ECMM).

Alida Fe Talento M.D., FRCPath, FFPath, FRCPI is Consultant Microbiologist at the Department of Microbiology of the Children's Health Ireland at Temple St. Dublin and Honorary Senior Clinical Lecturer of the Department of Microbiology Royal College of Surgeons, Ireland. She obtained her Doctor of Medicine degree from the University of Dublin, Trinity College, in 2017 with her dissertation on the epidemiology, diagnosis, and management of invasive fungal diseases in patients requiring critical care. Her research interests are fungal diagnostics, antifungal resistance, and antifungal stewardship. She currently is Secretary of the Irish Fungal Society and Council Member of the European Confederation of Medical Mycology.

Journal of *Fungi*

MDPI

Editorial

Fungal Infections Complicating COVID-19: With the Rain Comes the Spores

Alida Fe Talento [1,*] and Martin Hoenigl [2,3,4,*]

1 Department of Microbiology, Children's Health Ireland at Temple St., D01 YC67 Dublin, Ireland
2 Division of Infectious Diseases and Global Health, University of California San Diego, San Diego, CA 92093, USA
3 Clinical and Translational Fungal-Working Group, University of California San Diego, San Diego, CA 92093, USA
4 Section of Infectious Diseases and Tropical Medicine, Medical University of Graz, 8036 Graz, Austria
* Correspondence: talenta@tcd.ie (A.F.T.); hoeniglmartin@gmail.com (M.H.)

Received: 5 November 2020; Accepted: 10 November 2020; Published: 11 November 2020

Within the last 12 months, coronavirus disease 2019 (COVID-19) caused by the severe acute respiratory syndrome coronavirus-2 (SARS-CoV-2) spread globally to pandemic proportions. Although the majority of cases have asymptomatic or mild infections, a significant proportion progress to severe pneumonia and acute respiratory distress syndrome requiring critical care. Opportunistic infections following severe respiratory viral infections have been recognized since the 1918 influenza pandemic. Among critically ill patients with COVID-19, particularly secondary fungal infections caused by *Aspergillus* and *Candida* spp. are increasingly described. We, therefore, hosted a Special Issue focusing on fungal infections complicating COVID-19 and are delighted that a total of seven high quality papers were published within this issue. COVID-19-associated pulmonary aspergillosis (CAPA) has been reviewed in detail by Arastehfar et al., where authors have also shed light on the immunopathogenesis of CAPA, which is believed to occur due to a defective immune response in patients with severe COVID-19 leading to a hyperimmune state and dysfunctional T-lymphocytes infections [1]. The release of danger-associated molecular patterns during severe COVID-19 may contribute to pulmonary epithelial damage; collateral effects of host recognition pathways required for the activation of antiviral immunity may, paradoxically, contribute to a highly permissive inflammatory environment that favours the development of pulmonary mould infections [1]. CAPA has been shown to be associated with increased mortality that can only be lowered by early initiation of antifungal treatment [2,3]; thus, early diagnosis is essential. Mohamed et al. suggest screening patients with severe COVID-19 in intensive care who remain unwell using a combination of fungal biomarkers which include culture and galactomannan of deep respiratory samples, serum galactomannan and 1-3 beta-d-glucan, and molecular assays as well as computerised tomography [4]. Gangneux et al. demonstrated that molecular assays to detect Aspergillus DNA from blood and respiratory samples resulted in higher sensitivity when compared to culture based methods which may aid in the early diagnosis of CAPA [5]. Future studies should evaluate the role of point-of-care diagnostics for the diagnosis of CAPA, such as the Aspergillus Lateral Flow Device assay, which has shown promise for diagnosing pulmonary aspergillosis in the critical care setting [6].

Importantly, there are also reports of yeast infections in critically ill patients with COVID-19. While Arastehfar et al. point out that—in contrast to CAPA—there is no immunological predisposition, *Candida* blood stream infections may occur in patients with classical clinical risk factors including long-term ICU stays, indwelling vascular devices, and receipt of antibiotics and corticosteroids [7]. In another report in this Special Issue, two patients developed *Saccharomyces* blood stream infection after receipt of probiotics supplementation which contained the same strain of this yeast while in critical care [8], highlighting the risk of fungal translocation in these severely ill patients.

Lastly, but equally important, is the early initiation of appropriate antifungal therapy when secondary fungal infections are suspected. The global emergence of antifungal resistance in the two major fungal pathogens has made treatment more challenging given that there are only a few classes of systemic antifungal agents. Meijer et al. report on the first published case of CAPA due to a triazole-resistant *A. fumigatus* [9], while Posteraro et al. presents a case of a pan-echinocandin resistant *C. glabrata* bloodstream infection [10], with both cases leading to a fatal outcome. These cases underline the importance of performing antifungal susceptibility testing and antifungal stewardship.

As the global pandemic continues, we cannot overemphasise the need for a low threshold to screen for fungal infections for early diagnosis and allow appropriate antifungal therapy. Again, we express our sincere thanks to the authors and reviewers for their contribution to the literature on this very important topic, despite their busy schedules taking care of these patients with COVID-19.

Conflicts of Interest: A.F.T. received research funding and personal fees from Gilead and Pfizer. M.H. received research funding from Gilead, Pfizer and Astellas.

References

1. Arastehfar, A.; Carvalho, A.; Veerdonk, F.L. Van De COVID-19 Associated Pulmonary Aspergillosis (CAPA)—From Immunology to Treatment. *J. Fungi* **2020**, *6*, 91. [CrossRef] [PubMed]
2. Hoenigl, M. Invasive Fungal Disease complicating COVID-19: When it rains it pours. *Clin. Infect. Dis.* **2020**. [CrossRef]
3. White, L.; Dhillon, R.; Cordey, A.; Hughes, H.; Faggian, F.; Soni, S.; Pandey, M.; Whitaker, H.; May, A.; Morgan, M.; et al. A National Strategy to Diagnose COVID-19 Associated Invasive Fungal Disease in the ICU. *Clin. Infect. Dis.* **2020**. [CrossRef]
4. Mohamed, A.; Rogers, T.R.; Talento, A.F. COVID-19 Associated Invasive Pulmonary Aspergillosis: Diagnostic and Therapeutic Challenges. *J. Fungi* **2020**, *6*, 115. [CrossRef] [PubMed]
5. Gangneux, J.-P.; Reizine, F.; Guegan, H.; Pinceaux, K.; Le Balch, P.; Prat, E.; Pelletier, R.; Belaz, S.; Le Souhaitier, M.; Le Tulzo, Y.; et al. Is the COVID-19 Pandemic a Good Time to Include *Aspergillus* Molecular Detection to Categorize Aspergillosis in ICU Patients? A Monocentric Experience. *J. Fungi* **2020**, *6*, 105. [CrossRef] [PubMed]
6. Jenks, J.D.; Prattes, J.; Frank, J.; Spiess, B.; Mehta, S.R.; Boch, T.; Buchheidt, D.; Hoenigl, M. Performance of the Bronchoalveolar Lavage Fluid Aspergillus Galactomannan Lateral Flow Assay with Cube Reader for Diagnosis of Invasive Pulmonary Aspergillosis: A Multicenter Cohort Study. *Clin. Infect. Dis.* **2020**. [CrossRef] [PubMed]
7. Arastehfar, A.; Carvalho, A.A.R.; Nguyen, M.H.; Hedayati, M.T.; Netea, M.G.; Perlin, D.S.; Hoenigl, M. COVID-19-Associated Candidiasis (CAC): An Underestimated Complication in the Absence of Immunological Predispositions? *J. Fungi* **2020**, *6*, 211. [CrossRef] [PubMed]
8. Ventoulis, I.; Sarmourli, T.; Amoiridou, P.; Mantzana, P.; Exindari, M.; Gioula, G.; Vyzantiadis, T. Bloodstream Infection by *Saccharomyces cerevisiae* in Two COVID-19 Patients after Receiving Supplementation of *Saccharomyces* in the ICU. *J. Fungi* **2020**, *6*, 98. [CrossRef] [PubMed]
9. Meijer, E.F.J.; Dofferhoff, A.S.M.; Hoiting, O.; Buil, J.B.; Meis, J.F. Azole-Resistant COVID-19-Associated Pulmonary Aspergillosis in an Immunocompetent Host: A Case Report. *J. Fungi* **2020**, *6*, 79. [CrossRef] [PubMed]
10. Posteraro, B.; Torelli, R.; Vella, A.; Leone, P.M.; De Angelis, G.; De Carolis, E.; Ventura, G.; Sanguinetti, M.; Fantoni, M. Pan-Echinocandin-Resistant *Candida glabrata* Bloodstream Infection Complicating COVID-19: A Fatal Case Report. *J. Fungi* **2020**, *6*, 163. [CrossRef] [PubMed]

Publisher's Note: MDPI stays neutral with regard to jurisdictional claims in published maps and institutional affiliations.

Journal of *Fungi*

MDPI

Review

COVID-19 Associated Pulmonary Aspergillosis (CAPA)—From Immunology to Treatment

Amir Arastehfar [1,*,†], Agostinho Carvalho [2,3,*,†], Frank L. van de Veerdonk [4,5], Jeffrey D. Jenks [6,7], Philipp Koehler [8,9], Robert Krause [10], Oliver A. Cornely [8,9,11,12], David S. Perlin [1], Cornelia Lass-Flörl [13] and Martin Hoenigl [7,10,14,*,†] on behalf of the ECMM Working Group Immunologic Markers for Treatment Monitoring and Diagnosis in Invasive Mold Infection

1 Center for Discovery and Innovation, Hackensack Meridian Health, Nutley, NJ 07110, USA; david.perlin@hmh-cdi.org
2 Life and Health Sciences Research Institute (ICVS), School of Medicine, University of Minho, 4710-057 Braga, Portugal
3 ICVS/3B's—PT Government Associate Laboratory, 4710-057 Braga, Portugal
4 Department of Internal Medicine, Radboud University Medical Center, 6525 Nijmegen, The Netherlands; frank.vandeveerdonk@radboudumc.nl
5 Radboud Institute of Molecular Life Sciences, Radboud University Medical Center, 6525 Nijmegen, The Netherlands
6 Department of Medicine, University of California San Diego, San Diego, CA 92103, USA; jjenks@ucsd.edu
7 Clinical and Translational Fungal-Working Group, University of California San Diego, La Jolla, CA 92093, USA
8 Department I of Internal Medicine, Medical Faculty and University Hospital Cologne, University of Cologne, 50937 Cologne, Germany; philipp.koehler@uk-koeln.de (P.K.); oliver.cornely@uk-koeln.de (O.A.C.)
9 Cologne Excellence Cluster on Cellular Stress Responses in Aging-Associated Diseases (CECAD), University of Cologne, 50937 Cologne, Germany
10 Section of Infectious Diseases and Tropical Medicine, Department of Internal Medicine, Medical University of Graz, 8036 Graz, Austria; Robert.krause@medunigraz.at
11 Zentrum fuer klinische Studien (ZKS) Köln, Clinical Trials Centre Cologne, 50937 Cologne, Germany
12 German Center for Infection Research (DZIF), Partner Site Bonn-Cologne, Medical Faculty and University Hospital Cologne, University of Cologne, 50937 Cologne, Germany
13 Division of Hygiene and Medical Microbiology, Medical University of Innsbruck, 6020 Innsbruck, Austria; cornelia.lass-floerl@i-med.ac.at
14 Division of Infectious Diseases and Global Public Health, Department of Medicine, University of California, San Diego, San Diego, CA 92093, USA
* Correspondence: a.arastehfar.nl@gmail.com (A.A.); agostinhocarvalho@med.uminho.pt (A.C.); hoeniglmartin@gmail.com (M.H.); Tel.: +1-201-880-3100 (A.A.); +351-253-604811 (A.C.); +1-619-543-5605 (M.H.); Fax: +1-201-880-3100 (A.A.); +351-253-604811 (A.C.); +1-619-543-5605 (M.H.)
† These authors contributed equally to this work.

Received: 5 June 2020; Accepted: 22 June 2020; Published: 24 June 2020

Abstract: Like severe influenza, coronavirus disease-19 (COVID-19) resulting in acute respiratory distress syndrome (ARDS) has emerged as an important disease that predisposes patients to secondary pulmonary aspergillosis, with 35 cases of COVID-19 associated pulmonary aspergillosis (CAPA) published until June 2020. The release of danger-associated molecular patterns during severe COVID-19 results in both pulmonary epithelial damage and inflammatory disease, which are predisposing risk factors for pulmonary aspergillosis. Moreover, collateral effects of host recognition pathways required for the activation of antiviral immunity may, paradoxically, contribute to a highly permissive inflammatory environment that favors fungal pathogenesis. Diagnosis of CAPA remains challenging, mainly because bronchoalveolar lavage fluid galactomannan testing and culture, which represent the most sensitive diagnostic tests for aspergillosis in the ICU, are hindered by the fact that bronchoscopies are rarely performed in COVID-19 patients due to the risk of disease transmission. Similarly, autopsies are rarely performed, which may result in an underestimation of the prevalence of CAPA. Finally, the treatment of CAPA is complicated by drug–drug interactions associated with broad spectrum azoles, renal tropism and damage caused by SARS-CoV-2, which may challenge the use of liposomal amphotericin B, as well as the emergence of azole-resistance. This clinical reality creates an urgency for new antifungal drugs currently in advanced clinical development with more promising pharmacokinetic and pharmacodynamic profiles.

Keywords: SARS COV-2; *Aspergillus*; novel coronavirus; superinfection; co-infection; risk factors; prevalence; challenges; immune response; expert statement; European Confederation of Medical Mycology

1. Introduction

Invasive fungal infections caused by various fungal genera, including *Aspergillus*, complicate and endanger lives of millions of individuals annually [1]. *Aspergillus* genera, most frequently *Aspergillus fumigatus*, are ubiquitous in the environment and cause a wide range of infections in humans, including invasive pulmonary aspergillosis (IPA), chronic pulmonary aspergillosis (CPA), allergic bronchopulmonary aspergillosis (ABPA), chronic rhinosinusitis, fungal asthma, and *Aspergillus* bronchitis [2,3]. IPA, the most severe manifestation of disease from *Aspergillus*, is associated with high mortality rates and is a prominent complication among those with profound immunosuppression, such as those undergoing hematopoietic transplantation, as well as those with structural lung damage who receive systemic corticosteroids for their underlying condition, such as patients with chronic obstructive pulmonary diseases (COPD) [2].

Recently, it has been reported that a relatively high number of influenza patients presenting with severe acute respiratory distress syndrome (ARDS) also rapidly develop IPA, which is associated with increased duration of hospitalization and mortality [4,5]. Corticosteroid use and pulmonary epithelial damages caused by severe influenza are the main risk factors for developing IPA [4,5]. The recent global pandemic of coronavirus disease-19, also known as COVID-19, has infected over 6 million patients worldwide, with more than 360,000 deaths. It has been shown that up to 40% of COVID-19 hospitalized patients can develop ARDS [6], and thereby become susceptible to acquire co-infections caused by bacteria and also *Aspergillus* spp. [7,8], although frequency of co-infections seems to vary between centers and overall co-infections may occur less frequently than with severe influenza [9]. Once they occur, these superinfections are associated with high mortality rates and may prolong the acute phase of COVID-19 [10]. In this comprehensive review, we discuss various aspects of COVID-19 associated pulmonary aspergillosis (CAPA), focusing specifically on immunology, risk factors, prevalence, diagnosis, treatment, and current challenges.

2. Immunology

Dissecting the complex pathogenesis of CAPA requires a molecular understanding of the physiological processes whereby infection with SARS-CoV-2 facilitates fungal pathogenesis. Similar to other SARS coronaviruses, SARS-CoV-2 targets and invades epithelial cells and type II pneumocytes through binding of the SARS spike protein to the angiotensin-converting enzyme 2 (ACE2) receptors [11]. Cleavage of the S1/S2 domain by the type 2 transmembrane protease TMPRSS2 leads to the activation of the spike protein [12], thereby facilitating viral entry into the target cell via ACE2. Besides its role as a SARS virus receptor, ACE2 was also demonstrated to be required for protection from severe acute lung injury in ARDS [13]. In support of this, an insertion/deletion polymorphism that affects ACE activity was associated with ARDS susceptibility and outcome [14]. Whether the preceding interaction of SARS-CoV-2 with host cells, by disrupting the regulation of the renin-angiotensin system and or the kallikrein-kinin system, contributes to the development of CAPA, is not known.

Viral entry and infection elicit an immune response, which is initiated by the establishment of an inflammatory cascade by innate immune cells. Although the receptor(s) and signaling pathways involved in the immune recognition of *Aspergillus* and the downstream production of inflammatory mediators are relatively well characterized [15], not much is known regarding how the immune system senses and responds to SARS-CoV-2. Based on the available knowledge for infections with other coronaviruses, two possible mechanisms can be anticipated and are likely to explain the development of ARDS and consequently CAPA. The first involves the release of danger-associated molecular patterns (DAMPs), signal molecules released by dying or damaged cells that act as endogenous danger signals to promote and exacerbate the immune and inflammatory response leading to lung injury [16]. It is noteworthy that DAMPs have also been shown to regulate inflammation in fungal diseases [17]. The DAMP/receptor for advanced glycation end-products axis was found to integrate with Toll-like receptors (TLRs) to generate and amplify the inflammatory response in experimental aspergillosis [18]. Moreover, recipients of allogeneic stem-cell transplantation harboring genetic variants underlying a hyperactivation of danger signaling in response to infection displayed an increased risk of developing IPA [19]. This emerging concept could help explain fungal pathogenesis in conditions of exuberant inflammation such as that observed in COVID-19 patients and highlights DAMP targeting as potential immunomodulatory strategy in CAPA.

A second possibility involves the collateral effects of recognition pathways required for the activation of antiviral immunity that may, paradoxically, contribute to an inflammatory environment that favors secondary infections. ACE2 is not well expressed on immune cells and SARS-CoV are recognized by TLR4 and TLR3, leading to the activation of MyD88- or TRIF-mediated signaling, respectively [20,21]. Of note, this may be potentiated in the presence of *Aspergillus spp.* which activate TLR4/MyD88/TRIF through the cleavage of fibrinogen [22]. It is likely that SARS-CoV-2 may elicit, to a large extent, overlapping signaling pathways towards the production of inflammatory cytokines. In addition, the activation of the inflammasome by SARS-CoV and the consequent production of IL-1β is an event that contributes further to the hyperinflammatory response [23]. A transcriptome analysis of COVID-19 patients revealed an early immune response characterized by a marked upregulation of the IL-1 pathway, even after respiratory function nadir [24]. The possibility that IL-1 and related pro-inflammatory pathways could serve as therapeutic targets was demonstrated by the favorable responses in severe COVID-19 patients with secondary hemophagocytic lymphohistiocytosis treated with the interleukin-1 receptor antagonist anakinra [25]. Similar findings were also disclosed in acute leukemia patients with COVID-19 [26]. Likewise, IL-1 blockade with anakinra has also been found to ameliorate inflammation in both chronic granulomatous disease [27] and cystic fibrosis [28], and in either case, to restrain susceptibility to infection or colonization by *Aspergillus*. Therefore, the early hyperactivation of the IL-1 pathway induced by the SARS-CoV-2 infection may be a major factor establishing a highly permissive inflammatory environment that favors fungal pathogenesis.

Besides IL-1, increased levels of IL-6 have also been consistently reported in severe cases of COVID-19 [29,30], with an impact on immune cell function and the anti-viral mechanisms of immune cells [31]. An enhanced production of IL-6 is also observed in epithelial cells following infection with *A. fumigatus*, suggesting that, at least in some patients, the co-infection may contribute to the increased levels of this cytokine in severe COVID-19 patients [32]. In a large patient series of COVID-19 patients with ARDS, the use of the IL-6 receptor antagonist tocilizumab was recently reported to promote rapid and sustained responses associated with significant clinical improvement [33]. However, such clinical approach could paradoxically enhance the predisposition to CAPA, similar to animal models of IL-6 deficiency subjected to experimental aspergillosis [34]. For this reason, ongoing trials are addressing the combined use of IL-6 antagonists and antifungal prophylaxis in severe COVID-19 patients.

An emerging body of evidence supports therefore an increased systemic inflammatory reaction in patients with severe SARS-CoV-2 infection who are more likely to develop CAPA. In this regard, increased levels of circulating proinflammatory cytokines, such as TNF, were observed in patients requiring intensive care, compared to those with milder infections [35]. Other studies, however, have also unveiled marked defects in immune cell populations, namely T-lymphocytes, as another factor explaining the immune dysfunction in patients with COVID-19 [36]. This suggests that while sustained innate immune function leads to hyperinflammation [37], lymphocyte numbers decline, and their function may be defective. In this regard, severe lymphocytopenia was among the factors in a risk score model that predicted the development of invasive mold disease in patients with hematological malignances [38]. It is thus reasonable to speculate that in elderly individuals or with co-morbidities, defective immune responses to SARS-CoV-2 may allow unrestricted viral replication which, in turn, elicits hyperinflammation and severe complications such as ARDS [39], besides establishing favorable conditions for the acquisition of secondary infections, such as CAPA.

While there is much to be learned about CAPA, our current understanding of the pathophysiology of other coinfections with respiratory viruses such as influenza [40] provides an important framework towards the effective design of immunotherapeutic approaches and the identification of the patients that could benefit the most from them.

3. Risk Factors Implicated in CAPA Development

Importantly, the pathogenesis of IPA differs between neutropenic and non-neutropenic patients, including those with COVID-19, impacting clinical presentation, radiological findings and diagnostic test results in the mycology laboratory [41,42]. Despite these important differences, revised European Organization for Research and Treatment of Cancer/Invasive Fungal Infections Cooperative Group and National Institute of Allergy and Infectious Diseases Mycoses Study Group (EORTC/MSG) definitions [43] focus primarily on neutropenic patients with underlying hematological malignancies and "typical" presentation of IPA and have been shown to have limited applicability and inferior performance in non-neutropenic patients who frequently do not fulfil radiological and host criteria, including patients with COVID-19 [41,44]. This has resulted in the creation of an alternative clinical algorithm for diagnosing IPA in the ICU setting in 2012 [41], which defines putative IPA and is now the standard of care for defining IPA in the ICU [4,45], where highly reliable definitions of IA are still missing (work on improved definitions is currently in progress [45,46]).

Rapid development of CAPA few days following ICU admission [47] resembles the observation made for influenza-associated pulmonary aspergillosis [4,5]. Risk factors predisposing COVID-19 patients to develop secondary pulmonary aspergillosis are similar to those identified for influenza-IPA superinfections [4,5]. The most important risk factors include severe lung damage during the course of COVID-19 [48], the use of corticosteroids in those with ARDS, the widespread use of broad-spectrum antibiotics in intensive care units [49], and the presence of comorbidities such as structural lung defects [47,50–52].

There are some reports revealing that pulmonary fibrosis can be triggered by the cytokine storm activated by the viral antigens, toxicity posed by drugs, high airway pressure and hypoxia-induced acute lung injury secondary to mechanical ventilation [53]. While interstitial pulmonary fibrosis per se does not predispose to development of IPA, a small subset of these COVID-19 survivors may require long term corticosteroid treatment, which may predispose them to CAPA years after the acute phase of the viral infection. Overall, 29% of the CAPA cases published to date (10/35) had received systemic corticosteroids (Table 1). In those with ARDS, systemic corticosteroids are used to alleviate the immune responses and prevent cytokine storm [6,54–56], but may at the same time increase vulnerability for developing secondary infections [4,5].

Table 1. Clinical characteristics of COVID-19 patients with pulmonary aspergillosis published before 10 June 2020.

Country (Prevalence) COHORT [Ref]	Age/Sex	Underlying Conditions	CAPA Classification	Local/Systemic Corticosteroid Use	GM (ODI)/Serum BDG (pg/mL)/qPCR	Species (Voriconazole Susceptibility Pattern)	Treatment #	Outcome
Germany (5/19; 26.3%) ARDS [50]	62/F	Cholecystectomy for cholecystitis, arterial hypertension, obesity with sleep apnea, hypercholesterolemia, ex-smoker, COPD (GOLD 2)	Putative	Inhaled steroids for COPD	GM Serum negative GM BALF> 2.5 qPCR BALF = Positive	*Aspergillus fumigatus* (S) culture from BALF	VCZ	Died
	70/M	Vertebral disc prolapse left L4/5, flavectomy and nucleotomy, Ex-smoker	Putative	No	GM Serum = 0.7 GM BALF> 2.5 qPCR BALF = Positive	*A. fumigatus* by PCR; negative culture	ISA	Died
	54/M	Arterial hypertension, diabetes mellitus, aneurysm coiling right *A. vertebralis*	Putative	Intravenous corticosteroid therapy 0.4 mg/kg/d, total of 13 days)	GM Serum negative GM BALF> 2.5 qPCR BALF = Positive	*A. fumigatus* (S) culture from tracheal aspirate	CASPO→ VCZ	Alive
	73/M	Arterial hypertension, bullous emphysema, smoker, COPD (GOLD 3), Previous Hepatitis B	Putative	Inhaled steroids for COPD	GM Serum negative qPCR tracheal secretion = Positive	*A. fumigatus* (S) culture from tracheal aspirate	VCZ	Died
	54/F	None	Putative	No	GM Serum = 1.3 and 2.7 qPCR tracheal secretion = Negative	Negative culture	CASPO→ VCZ	Alive
France (9/27; 33.3%) ARDS * [51]	53/M	Hypertension, obesity, ischemic heart disease	Putative	Dexamethasone iv 20 mg once daily from day 1 to day 5, followed by 10 mg once daily from day 6 to day 10	GM Serum = 0.13 GM BALF = 0.89 BDG = 523 qPCR = Negative	Negative culture	None	Alive
	59/F	Hypertension, obesity, diabetes	Putative	No	GM Serum = 0.04 GM BALF = 0.03 qPCR = Negative	*A. fumigatus*, culture from BALF	None	Alive
	69/F	Hypertension, obesity	Putative	Dexamethasone iv 20 mg once daily from day 1 to day 5, followed by 10 mg once daily from day 6 to day 10	GM Serum = 0.04 BDG = 7.8 qPCR BALF = 23.9	*A. fumigatus*, culture from tracheal secretion	None	Alive
	63/F	Hypertension, diabetes, ischemic heart disease	Putative	Dexamethasone iv 20 mg once daily from day 1 to day 5, followed by 10 mg once daily from day 6 to day 10	GM Serum = 0.51 GM BALF = 0.15 BDG = 63	Negative culture	None	Died
	43/M	Asthma with steroid use history	Putative	No	GM Serum = 0.04 GM BALF = 0.12 BDG = 7 qPCR = Negative	*A. fumigatus*, culture from BALF	None	Alive
	79/M	Hypertension	Putative	Dexamethasone iv 20 mg once daily from day 1 to day 5, followed by 10 mg once daily from day 6 to day 10	GM Serum = 0.02 GM BALF = 0.05 BDG = 23 qPCR BALF = 34.5	*A. fumigatus*, culture from BALF	None	Alive

Table 1. *Cont.*

Country (Prevalence) COHORT [Ref]	Age/Sex	Underlying Conditions	CAPA Classification	Local/Systemic Corticosteroid Use	GM (ODI)/Serum BDG (pg/mL)/qPCR	Species (Voriconazole Susceptibility Pattern)	Treatment #	Outcome
	77/M	Hypertension, asthma	Putative	Dexamethasone iv 20 mg once daily from day 1 to day 5, followed by 10 mg once daily from day 6 to day 10	GM Serum = 0.37 GM BALF = 3.91 BDG = 135 qPCR BALF = 29	*A. fumigatus*, culture from BALF	VCZ	Died
	75/F	Hypertension, diabetes	Putative	Dexamethasone iv 20 mg once daily from day 1 to day 5, followed by 10 mg once daily from day 6 to day 10	GM Serum = 0.37 GM BALF = 0.36 BDG = 450 qPCR BALF = 31.7	*A. fumigatus*, culture from BALF	CASPO	Died
	47/M	Multiple myeloma with steroid therapy	Probable	No	GM Serum = 0.09 BDG = 14	*A. fumigatus*, culture from tracheal secretion	None	Died
Netherlands (6/31; 19.4%)ARDS [47]	83/M	Cardiomyopathy	Possible	Prednisolone 0·13 mg/kg/day for 28 days pre-admission	GM Serum = 0.4	*A. fumigatus*, culture from tracheal aspirate	VCZ + ANID (5/6) L-AmB (1/6)	Died
	67/M	COPD (GOLD 3), Post RTx NSCLC 2014	Possible	Prednisolone 0·37 mg/kg/day for 2 days pre-admission	NA	*A. fumigatus*, culture from tracheal aspirate		Died
	75/M	COPD (GOLD 2a)	Probable	No	GM BALF = 4.0	*A. fumigatus*, culture from BALF		Died
	43/M	None	Probable	No	GM Serum = 0.1 GM BALF = 3.8	NA		Alive
	57/M	Bronchial asthma	Probable	Fluticasone 1·94 mcg/kg/day for 1 month pre-admission	GM Serum = 0.1 GM BALF = 1.6	*A. fumigatus*. culture from BALF		Died
	58/M	None	Possible	No	NA	*Aspergillus spp.* (S), culture from sputum		Alive
Belgium (7/20; 35%)ARDS [52]	86/M	Hypercholesterinemia	NA	No	GM serum = 0.1	*A. flavus* culture from tracheal aspirate	None	Died
	38/M	Obesity, hypercholesterinemia	Proven	No	GM serum = 0.3 GM BALF > 2.8	*A. fumigatus* culture from BALF	VCZ, ISA	Alive
	62/M	Diabetes	Proven	No	GM serum = 0.2 GM BALF = 2	*A. fumigatus* culture from BALF	VCZ	Died
	73/M	Diabetes, obesity, hypertension, hypercholesterinemia	Proven	No	GM serum= 0.1 GM BALF > 2.8	*A. fumigatus* culture from BALF	VCZ	Alive
	77/M	Diabetes, chronic kidney disease, hypertension, pemphigus foliaceus	Proven	Yes, ND	GM serum = 0.1 GM BALF = 2.79	*A. fumigatus* culture from BALF	VCZ	Alive
	55/M	HIV, hypertension, hypercholesterinemia	NA	No	GM serum = 0.80 GM BALF = 0.69	Negative culture	VCZ, ISA	Died
	75/M	Acute myeloid leukemia	NA	No	GM BALF = 2.63	*A. fumigatus* culture from BALF	VCZ	Died

Table 1. *Cont.*

Country (Prevalence) COHORT [Ref]	Age/Sex	Underlying Conditions	CAPA Classification	Local/Systemic Corticosteroid Use	GM (ODI)/Serum BDG (pg/mL)/qPCR	Species (Voriconazole Susceptibility Pattern)	Treatment #	Outcome
France (1) ARDS [57]	74/M	Myelodysplastic syndrome, CD8 + T-cell lymphocytosis, Hashimoto's thyroiditis, hypertension, benign prostatic hypertrophy	Putative	No	First GM on tracheal secretion = Negative First qPCR = Positive Second GM tracheal secretion = NA Second qPCR = Positive Direct smear of the second sample = branched septate hyphae	*A. fumigatus*, culture of the second tracheal secretion	None	Died
France (1/5; 20%) Mixed ICU [58]	80/M	Thyroid cancer (patient presented with ARDS)	Putative	NA	No	*A. flavus*, culture from tracheal secretion	VCZ→ ISA	Died
Italy (1) ARDS [59]	73/M	Diabetes, hypertension, obesity, hyperthyroidism, atrial fibrillation	Proven	No	GM Serum = 8.6 qPCR from paraffin block tissue = Positive	*A. fumigatus*, culture from BALF	L-AmB → ISA	Died
Austria (1) ARDS [60]	70/M	COPD (GOLD 2), obstructive sleep apnea syndrome, insulin-dependent type 2 diabetes with end organ damage, arterial hypertension, coronary heart disease, and obesity	Putative	Inhaled Budesonide (400 mg per day)	GM Serum = Negative BDG = Negative LFD Positive from endotracheal aspiration	*A. fumigatus*, culture from endotracheal aspiration	VCZ	Died
Germany (2) ARDS [61]	80/M	Suspected pulmonary fibrosis	ND	No	GM Serum = 1.5 GM BALF = 6.3	*A. fumigatus*, culture from BALF	L-AmB	Died
	70/M	None	ND	No	GM Serum = Negative GM BALF = 6.1	*A. fumigatus*, culture from BALF	L-AmB	Died
Netherlands (1) ARDS [62]	74/F	Polyarthritis, reflux, stopped smoking 20 years ago	Putative	No	GM serum = Persistently < 0.5 GM tracheal aspirate = >3 BDG serum = 1590	*A. fumigatus*, culture from tracheal aspirate (R) $^{TR34/L98H}$ ICZ = 16µg/mL, VCZ = 2µg/mL, and POSA = 0.5µg/ml	VCZ + CASPO→ Oral VCZ→ L-AmB	Died
Australia (1) ARDS [63]	66/F	Hypertension, osteopenia, ex-smoker (20 pack years)	Putative	No	N/A	*A. fumigatus* culture from tracheal aspirate (3x)	VCZ + Therapeutic Drug monitoring	Alive

* All serum qPCR remained negative. # All dosages are standard dosages (e.g., VCZ 6 mg/kg bid Day 1, and 4 mg/kg bid starting Day 2) [64]. ARDS: acute respiratory distress syndrome; NA: not applicable; ND: not determined; BALF: bronchoalveolar lavage fluid; BDG: beta-D-Glucan; COPD: chronic obstructive pulmonary disease; GM; galactomannan; GOLD: global initiative for chronic obstructive lung disease; NSCLC: non-small-cell lung cancer; ODI: optical density index; RTx: radio therapy; LFD: lateral flow device; qPCR: quantitative real-time PCR; VCZ: voriconazole; ISA: isavuconazole; CASPO: caspofungin; ANID: anidulafungin; L-AmB: liposomal amphotericin B; ICZ: itraconazole; POSA = posaconazole.

Although detailed case series have not reported on antibiotic use among patients, broad-spectrum antibiotics are presumed to be used in 75% of COVID-19 patients admitted to ICU [49]. Since the human gut microbiome is a highly complicated structure of bacteria and fungi, although bacteria are the most diverse constituents, the administration of antibiotics results in perturbation of microbiome steady-state composition, which allows fungi to thrive, and may predispose the host to invasive fungal infections once the immune system becomes impaired [65,66].

Underlying medical conditions may also predispose COVID-19 patients to develop CAPA. Among the 35 CAPA cases published to date (Table 1), hypertension (17/35; 49%), diabetes (9/35; 26%), obesity (8/35; 23%), COPD (5/35; 14%), heart diseases (5/35; 14%), hypercholesterinemia (4/35; 11%), and asthma (3/35; 9%) were among the most prevalent comorbidities observed. While hypertension, coronary heart diseases, and diabetes increase the risk of infection overall [67–69], structural lung damage caused by COPD or asthma may particularly predispose patients to develop IPA [70].

4. CAPA Prevalence

Several studies from China reported high rates of *Aspergillus* infections among COVID-19 patients. In one study from the Jiangsu province in China, 60/257 COVID-19 (23.3%) patients had throat swab samples that tested positive for *Aspergillus* spp. and were reported as *Aspergillus* co-infections [8]. In another Chinese study from the Zhejiang province 8 of the 104 patients with COVID-19 (7.7%) patients were reported to have IPA although questions remain regarding criteria used for diagnosing IPA in this study (authors state EORTC/MSG criteria were used but all 8 patients seemingly lacked host factors) [71]. Another study from China reported that 27% of the COVID-19 patients (13/48) developed fungal infections but lacked further details [7]. In other reports from China, lower rates of fungal infections were reported ranging between 3.2–5% [54,55,72]. None of those studies have used specific definitions and standardized diagnostic algorithms to identify and define CAPA. In fact, diagnosis of pulmonary aspergillosis is challenging with culture exhibiting limited sensitivity [73,74], and galactomannan testing—the current gold standard—is rarely available in China [75]. As a result, some of these reported rates are likely an underestimate of the real burden of IPA in patients with COVID-19 requiring ICU admission, while other rates may be an overestimation due to potentially misinterpreting *Aspergillus* colonization in the upper respiratory tract as *Aspergillus* infection.

More recently, several studies and case-series from Europe (France, Germany, Belgium, and the Netherlands) have reported high rates of CAPA among COVID-19 cases with ARDS, ranging from 20–35% (Table 1) [47,50–52]. The development of CAPA was fairly rapid, with a median of 6 days and range of 3–28 days after ICU admission [47,52]. Moreover, two additional CAPA cases have been reported from Germany [61] and single cases have also been reported from the Netherlands [62], Austria [60], Italy [59], Australia [63], and France [57,58] (Table 1). Among 35 CAPA cases reported to date, there were a total of 5 proven cases [52,59]. The overall mortality rate was 63% (22/35), among whom 4 were female (4/8; 50%) and 14 were male (18/27; 67%). The mortality in case series reported from France, Germany, Belgium and Netherlands ranged between 44.5–66.7% [47,50–52]. Of particular importance was the 100% fatality rate of those with underlying diseases reported from the Netherlands, while the two patients without underlying conditions both survived [47]. Noteworthy is the fact that COVID-19 patients presented with ARDS typically fall into the elderly category [6], whereas ARDS in those infected with influenza involves both children <5 years old and elderly >65 years old [76]. The difficulties in diagnosing CAPA, which are outlined in more detail in the next section of this review, may also contribute to increased mortality rates. The most notable example is a study from France [57], where both culture and serology assays were negative for the initial respiratory samples and became only positive after the patient expired [57]. In a case from Italy, initial BALF culture was positive for *A. fumigatus* but the treatment was delayed for two days and only started after the serum galactomannan test became positive [59]. CAPA was later confirmed by autopsy examination [59]. As a result, authors encouraged prompt initiation of systemic antifungal therapy immediately after obtaining positive results even if *Aspergillus* is detected in samples from the upper respiratory tract [59]. Since azole resistance can be associated with a higher mortality rate when compared to patients infected with azole susceptible *A. fumigatus* isolates, it is of paramount importance to use antifungal susceptibility testing to inform targeted antifungal treatment, especially in regions with high azole resistance [77]. Azole-resistant *A. fumigatus* isolates were also persistently recovered from tracheal aspirates during the course of azole treatment in the most recent study from the Netherlands implicated a CAPA case for whom [62]. The azole-resistant *A. fumigatus* isolate (itraconazole, voriconazole, and posaconazole MICs were 16, 2, and 0.5 μg/mL, respectively) harbored a well-known mutation, TR34/L98H [62], presumed to have been acquired from the environment [77]. The in vitro MIC value of the isolate obtained at day 19 (2 mg/L) was higher than the voriconazole serum trough concentration measured on day 17 (1.43 mg/L) and despite switching voriconazole to L-AmB, the patient died due to deteriorating health conditions [62]. Overall, *A. fumigatus* appeared to be the most prevalent *Aspergillus* spp. isolated among respiratory samples with positive culture (26/29; 90%), followed by *A. flavus* (2/29; 7%).

5. Diagnostic Workup for Accurate Identification of CAPA

The optimal diagnostic algorithm for diagnosing CAPA is currently unknown, and this question is actively being investigated in an ongoing multinational explorative trial in conjunction with the European Confederation of Medical Mycology (ECMM). The most common methods to date include attempting to recover *Aspergillus spp.* on culture media of bronchoalveolar fluid (BALF) and tracheal aspirate, as well as utilizing serologic biomarker testing such as the conventional Galactomannan (GM) from BALF, tracheal aspirate, and serum specimens. Other diagnostic tests that may prove useful also include *Aspergillus* PCR, serum (1→3)-β-D-glucan (BDG), the *Aspergillus* galactomannan lateral flow assay (LFA) (IMMY, Norman, Oklahoma, USA), and the *Aspergillus*-specific lateral-flow device (LFD) test (OLM Diagnostics, Newcastle Upon Tyne, UK).

In published cases and case series from Germany [50,61], France [51,57,58], Italy [59], Austria [60], Belgium [52], Australia [63], and the Netherlands [47], CAPA was most commonly mycologically diagnosed by either culture from BALF or tracheal aspirate and/or based on a positive GM or LFD from BALF or tracheal aspirate (Table 1). Across published cases, *Aspergillus* culture was positive in 29/35 (83%) of patients; of those with a positive culture and a reported source, 16/29 (55%) were recovered from—often undirected—BALF, 12/29 (41%) from tracheal aspirate, and 1/29 (3%) from sputum. In those where a BALF GM test was performed, 14/23 (61%) had a titer ≥1.5 ODI and 16/23 (70%) a titer ≥0.5 ODI, while 6/28 (21%) of those with serum GM results had a titer > 0.5 ODI. PCR from respiratory specimens or tissue was positive in 10/14 (71%) and LFD from tracheal secretion positive in 1/1 of patients.

Thus, BALF and tracheal aspirate culture and conventional GM testing from BALF appear to be the most promising diagnostic modalities. Still, bronchoscopy can potentially aerosolize virus [78] in patients with COVID-19 infection, thus posing a risk to patients and personnel from SARS-CoV-2 virus. In many centers, the role of bronchoscopy is limited and testing from blood samples may be safer and more optimal and allow also for twice weekly screening which has been implemented in many centers [52], although the low levels of GM positivity from serum in these reports is discouraging, and the sensitivity of serum BDG, which is less specific for IA, was only 44% (4/9).

6. CAPA Treatment—Current Paradigm

While it is currently unknown whether antifungal treatment of COVID-19 associated IPA translates into a survival benefit, diagnosis should in most cases trigger early antifungal treatment. Outside the hematologic malignancy setting, voriconazole remains the recommended first-line treatment for IPA [79,80]. However, besides its narrow therapeutic window and the requirement for therapeutic drug monitoring to ensure efficacy and prevent neuro and hepatotoxicity [81], drug–drug interactions may particularly limit the use of voriconazole in the ICU setting [82]. Being metabolized via CYP2C19, CYP2C9, and CYP3A4, voriconazole is among the drugs most frequently associated with major drug–drug interactions in the ICU [83]. Furthermore, it may show interactions with experimental COVID-19 therapies, including hydroxychloroquine, atazanavir, lopinavir/ritonavir and last but not least—although weaker—with remdesivir, which is also a substrate for CYP3A4, although its metabolism is primarily mediated by hydrolase activity [84]. Isavuconazole and liposomal amphotericin B are the primary alternative options for treatment of IPA in the ICU [79]. Compared to voriconazole, isavuconazole shows a more favorable pharmacokinetic profile, and is associated with fewer toxicities. However, it is also metabolized via CYP3A4 and could therefore be problematic, although drug–drug interactions are generally less a problem with isavuconazole than with voriconazole [85,86]. Liposomal amphotericin B is a broadly effective alternative treatment option, however, in the ICU renal insufficiency often complicates initiation or requires discontinuation of this antifungal agent. This concern is particularly relevant for patients infected by SARS-CoV-2 which has shown renal tropism and been described as a frequent cause of kidney injury [87]. While itraconazole is now rarely used to treat invasive aspergillosis, it has been shown to exhibit some antiviral activity, specifically as a cholesterol transport inhibitor, and was effective in a feline coronavirus model [88]. In addition, its novel oral SUBA formulation has great bioavailability [89], and itraconazole may therefore be an alternative option for treating COVID-19 associated IPA, although it shares the problem of drug–drug interactions with other triazoles. While currently available echinocandins are not considered first-line treatment options for invasive aspergillosis due to their limited antifungal activity against *Aspergillus* spp., they are generally well tolerated with limited drug–drug interactions and show at least fungistatic activity against *Aspergillus* hyphae [90]. Furthermore, they synergistic interactions with some other antifungals, making them an excellent choice for combination antifungal therapy [90]. New antifungal classes currently under development, namely fosmanogepix and olorofim [91], may have equal efficacy without the same burden of drug–drug interactions and toxicity, and may therefore overcome the limitations of currently available antifungals and become the preferred treatment options in the near future. If the reported high incidence of COVID-19 associated IPA in ICU patients is confirmed in larger studies, there may be justification for prophylaxis trials, for which not only triazoles and nebulized liposomal amphotericin B [52], but also another novel antifungal currently under development, rezafungin (i.e., once weekly echinocandin with improved activity against *Aspergillus* spp.), may be a candidate [92].

7. The Current Challenges and How to Tackle Them

Bacterial, fungal and viral secondary infections or co-infections affect mortality. *Acinetobacter baumanii*, *Klebsiella pneumonia* and *Aspergillus* species are important nosocomial pathogens [93] complicating the disease course. Studies from France [51], Germany [50], Belgium [52], and the Netherlands [47], underline the role of CAPA. Diagnosing co-infections is complex and rapid diagnosis plays a crucial role in this setting [49]. Close monitoring for infection development is needed, as well as longitudinal sampling throughout the disease course using culture dependent and independent techniques. *Aspergillus* antigen and PCR testing of respiratory fluids should be a routine procedure for critically ill patients [94], specifically for those suffering from ARDS [50]. Co-infection with human metapneumovirus has been reported in two of five cases in the German CAPA series [50]. It is unknown whether hospitals caring for COVID-19 test comprehensive respiratory pathogen panels, and to date no analysis of mixed viral infection in COVID-19 patients has been reported. In the context of COVID-19, mixed viral infection may be misinterpreted as presence of innocent bystanders and thus remain underreported. With bronchoalveolar lavage and autopsy regarded as high-risk procedures, key diagnostic instruments are lacking. Autopsy studies are key to understanding pathophysiology of COVID-19 [95] and are critically enlighten interaction between SARS-CoV-2 and different pathogens. With availability of lower respiratory samples, normally obtained by BALF, the quality of microbiological and virological work up would be greatly improved. Inspection of trachea and bronchi is achieved by bronchoscopy, which is critical to find possible *Aspergillus* tracheobronchitis. Thus, physicians face the dilemma of taking the hazard of aerosolization of SARS-CoV-2, risking transmission versus the endeavor of facilitating the optimal diagnosis and treatment to the patients entrusted to their care.

To this day, our understanding of the true impact of *Aspergillus* co-infections remains frustratingly limited. Therefore, guidance on proper management of these high-risk procedures to prevent transmission and super spreading of SARS-CoV-2 is needed. The European Confederation of Medical Mycology initiated national multicenter studies aiming to explore the risk of fungal infections during COVID-19 [94] and is currently working on diagnostic and treatment algorithms. Key goals are to improve the outcome by avoiding misdiagnosis and by initiation of early and targeted antifungal treatment.

8. Future Perspectives

We anticipate that autopsies of COVID-19 fatalities will increase and likely prove the clinical relevance of CAPA [96]. Immune dysregulation together with epithelial lung damage stemming from COVID-19 immunopathology is a likely mechanism predisposing for IPA development [97]. IPA will be recognized as important co-infection in patients with severe COVID-19, but incidence will likely vary between different ICU settings. In settings where COVID-19 associated IPA occurs most commonly, screening for IPA in blood and true BALF samples (i.e., obtained via bronchoscopy) will be implemented followed by preemptive treatment in those with mycological evidence of IPA. In other high-incidence settings, clinical antifungal prophylaxis trials will be conducted among COVID-19 patients admitted to the ICU aiming to show a decrease in putative [4] and proven IPA cases, as well as overall mortality. Treatment trials will compare efficacy and safety of new antifungal drugs currently under development with established antifungals, initiating a new era of antifungal treatment.

Author Contributions: Conceptualization, M.H., A.A., and A.C.; writing—original draft preparation, A.A., A.C., M.H., F.L.v.d.V., J.D.J., C.L.-F., P.K., O.A.C., D.S.P., R.K.; writing—review and editing, M.H., A.A., A.C., F.L.v.d.V., J.D.J., C.L.-F., P.K., O.A.C., D.S.P., R.K. All authors have read and agreed to the published version of the manuscript.

Funding: AC was supported by the Fundação para a Ciência e a Tecnologia (FCT) (CEECIND/03628/2017, UIDB/50026/2020 and UIDP/50026/2020), and the Northern Portugal Regional Operational Programme (NORTE 2020), under the Portugal 2020 Partnership Agreement, through the European Regional Development Fund (ERDF) (NORTE-01-0145-FEDER-000013 and NORTE-01-0145-FEDER-000023). This research received no other external funding.

Conflicts of Interest: M.H. received research funding by Gilead and Pfizer. D.S.P. receives research support and/or serves on advisory boards for Amplyx, Cidara, Scynexis, N8 Medical, Merck, Regeneron, and Pfizer. P.K. has received non-financial scientific grants from Miltenyi Biotec GmbH, Bergisch Gladbach, Germany, and the Cologne Excellence Cluster on Cellular Stress Responses in Aging-Associated Diseases, University of Cologne, Cologne, Germany, and is an adivisor to, or received lecture honoraria from Akademie für Infektionsmedizin e.V., Astellas Pharma, Gilead Sciences, GPR Academy Ruesselsheim, MSD Sharp & Dohme GmbH, NOXXON Pharma NV., and University Hospital, LMU Munich outside the submitted work. O.A.C. is supported by the German Federal Ministry of Research and Education; is funded by the Deutsche Forschungsgemeinschaft (German Research Foundation) under Germany's Excellence Strategy (CECAD, EXC 2030 - 390661388); has received research grants from Actelion, Amplyx, Astellas, Basilea, Cidara, Da Volterra, F2G, Gilead, Janssen Pharmaceuticals, Medicines Company, MedPace, Melinta Therapeutics, MSD, Pfizer, and Scynexis; is a consultant to Actelion, Allecra Therapeutics, Amplyx, Astellas, Basilea, Biosys UK, Cidara, Da Volterra, Entasis, F2G, Gilead, Matinas, MedPace, Menarini Ricerche, Roche Diagnostics, MSD, Nabriva Therapeutics, Octapharma, Paratek Pharmaceuticals, Pfizer, PSI, Rempex, Scynexis, Seres Therapeutics, Tetraphase, and Vical; and received lecture honoraria from Astellas, Basilea, Gilead, Grupo Biotoscana, MSD, and Pfizer.

References

1. Brown, G.D.; Denning, D.W.; Gow, N.A.R.; Levitz, S.M.; Netea, M.G.; White, T.C. Hidden killers: Human fungal infections. *Sci. Transl. Med.* **2012**, *4*, 165rv13. [CrossRef] [PubMed]
2. Kosmidis, C.; Denning, D.W. The clinical spectrum of pulmonary aspergillosis. *Thorax* **2015**, *70*, 270–277. [CrossRef] [PubMed]
3. Li, E.; Knight, J.M.; Wu, Y.; Luong, A.; Rodriguez, A.; Kheradmand, F.; Corry, D.B. Airway mycosis in allergic airway disease. *Adv. Immunol.* **2019**, *142*, 85–140. [CrossRef]

4. Schauwvlieghe, A.F.A.D.; Rijnders, B.J.; Philips, N.; Verwijs, R.; Vanderbeke, L.; Van Tienen, C.; Lagrou, K.; Verweij, P.E.; Van De Veerdonk, F.L.; Gommers, D.; et al. Invasive aspergillosis in patients admitted to the intensive care unit with severe influenza: A retrospective cohort study. *Lancet Respir. Med.* **2018**, *6*, 782–792. [CrossRef]
5. Wauters, J.; Baar, I.; Meersseman, P.; Meersseman, W.; Dams, K.; De Paep, R.; Lagrou, K.; Wilmer, A.; Jorens, P.; Hermans, G. Invasive pulmonary aspergillosis is a frequent complication of critically ill H1N1 patients: A retrospective study. *Intensiv. Care Med.* **2012**, *38*, 1761–1768. [CrossRef] [PubMed]
6. Wu, C.; Chen, X.; Cai, Y.; Xia, J.; Zhou, X.; Xu, S.; Huang, H.; Zhang, L.; Zhou, X.; Du, C.; et al. Risk Factors Associated With Acute Respiratory Distress Syndrome and Death in Patients With Coronavirus Disease 2019 Pneumonia in Wuhan, China. *JAMA Intern. Med.* **2020**. [CrossRef]
7. Chen, X.; Zhao, B.; Qu, Y.; Chen, Y.; Xiong, J.; Feng, Y.; Men, D.; Huang, Q.; Liu, Y.; Yang, B.; et al. Detectable serum SARS-CoV-2 viral load (RNAaemia) is closely correlated with drastically elevated interleukin 6 (IL-6) level in critically ill COVID-19 patients. *Clin. Infect. Dis.* **2020**. [CrossRef]
8. Zhu, X.; Ge, Y.; Wu, T.; Zhao, K.; Chen, Y.; Wu, B.; Zhu, F.; Zhu, B.; Cui, L. Co-infection with respiratory pathogens among COVID-2019 cases. *Virus. Res.* **2020**, *11*, 198005. [CrossRef]
9. Rawson, T.M.; Moore, L.S.P.; Zhu, N.; Ranganathan, N.; Skolimowska, K.; Gilchrist, M.; Satta, G.; Cooke, G.; Holmes, A.H. Bacterial and fungal co-infection in individuals with coronavirus: A rapid review to support COVID-19 antimicrobial prescribing. *Clin. Infect. Dis.* **2020**. [CrossRef]
10. Lin, L.; Lu, L.; Cao, W.; Li, T. Hypothesis for potential pathogenesis of SARS- CoV-2 infection – A review of immune changes in patients with viral pneumonia. *Emerg. Microbes. Infect.* **2020**, *9*, 272–732. [CrossRef]
11. Kuba, K.; Imai, Y.; Rao, S.; Gao, H.; Guo, F.; Guan, B.; Huan, Y.; Yang, P.; Zhang, Y.; Deng, W.; et al. A crucial role of angiotensin converting enzyme 2 (ACE2) in SARS coronavirus–induced lung injury. *Nat. Med.* **2005**, *11*, 875–879. [CrossRef] [PubMed]
12. Glowacka, I.; Bertram, S.; Müller, M.A.; Allen, P.; Soilleux, E.; Pfefferle, S.; Steffen, I.; Tsegaye, T.S.; He, Y.; Gnirss, K.; et al. Evidence that TMPRSS2 Activates the Severe Acute Respiratory Syndrome Coronavirus Spike Protein for Membrane Fusion and Reduces Viral Control by the Humoral Immune Response. *J. Virol.* **2011**, *85*, 4122–4134. [CrossRef] [PubMed]
13. Imai, Y.; Kuba, K.; Rao, S.; Huan, Y.; Guo, F.; Guan, B.; Yang, P.; Sarao, R.; Wada, T.; Leong-Poi, H.; et al. Angiotensin-converting enzyme 2 protects from severe acute lung failure. *Nature* **2005**, *436*, 112–116. [CrossRef] [PubMed]
14. Marshall, R.P.; Webb, S.; Bellingan, G.J.; Montgomery, H.E.; Chaudhari, B.; McAnulty, R.J.; Humphries, S.E.; Hill, M.R.; Laurent, G.J. Angiotensin converting enzyme insertion/deletion polymorphism is associated with susceptibility and outcome in acute respiratory distress syndrome. *Am. J. Respir. Crit. Care Med.* **2002**, *166*, 646–650. [CrossRef]
15. Veerdonk, F.L.; Gresnigt, M.S.; Romani, L.; Netea, M.G.; Latge, J.P. *Aspergillus fumigatus* morphology and dynamic host interactions. *Nat. Rev. Microbiol.* **2017**, *15*, 661–674. [CrossRef]
16. Tolle, L.B.; Standiford, T.J. Danger-associated molecular patterns (DAMPs) in acute lung injury. *J. Pathol.* **2013**, *229*, 145–156. [CrossRef]
17. Cunha, C.; Carvalho, A.; Esposito, A.; Esposito, F.; Bistoni, F.; Romani, L. DAMP signaling in fungal infections and diseases. *Front. Immunol.* **2012**, *3*, 286. [CrossRef]
18. Sorci, G.; Giovannini, G.; Riuzzi, F.; Bonifazi, P.; Zelante, T.; Zagarella, S.; Bistoni, F.; Donato, R.; Romani, L. The danger signal S100B integrates pathogen- and danger-sensing pathways to restrain inflammation. *PLoS. Pathog.* **2011**, *7*, e1001315. [CrossRef]
19. Cunha, C.; Giovannini, G.; Pierini, A.; Bell, A.S.; Sorci, G.; Riuzzi, F.; Donato, R.; Rodrigues, F.; Velardi, A.; Aversa, F.; et al. Genetically-Determined Hyperfunction of the S100B/RAGE Axis Is a Risk Factor for Aspergillosis in Stem Cell Transplant Recipients. *PLoS ONE* **2011**, *6*, e27962. [CrossRef]
20. Totura, L.A.; Whitmore, A.; Agnihothram, S.; Schäfer, A.; Katze, M.G.; Heise, M.T.; Baric, R.S. Toll-like receptor 3 signaling via TRIF contributes to a protective innate immune response to severe acute respiratory syndrome coronavirus infection. *mBio* **2015**, *6*, e00638-15. [CrossRef]

21. Sheahan, T.; Morrison, T.E.; Funkhouser, W.; Uematsu, S.; Akira, S.; Baric, R.S.; Heise, M.T. MyD88 is required for protection from lethal infection with a mouse-adapted SARS-CoV. *PLoS. Pathog.* **2008**, *4*, e1000240. [CrossRef] [PubMed]
22. Millien, V.O.; Lu, W.; Shaw, J.; Yuan, X.; Mak, G.; Roberts, L.; Song, L.-Z.; Knight, J.M.; Creighton, C.J.; Luong, A.; et al. Cleavage of Fibrinogen by Proteinases Elicits Allergic Responses Through Toll-Like Receptor 4. *Science* **2013**, *341*, 792–796. [CrossRef]
23. Shi, C.S.; Nabar, N.R.; Huang, N.N.; Kehrl, J.H. SARS-Coronavirus open reading frame-8b triggers intracellular stress pathways and activates NLRP3 inflammasomes. *Cell. Death. Discov.* **2019**, *5*, 101. [CrossRef] [PubMed]
24. Ong, E.Z.; Chan, Y.F.Z.; Leong, W.Y.; Lee, N.M.Y.; Kalimuddin, S.; Mohideen, S.M.H.; Chan, K.S.; Tan, A.T.; Bertoletti, A.; Ooi, E.E.; et al. A Dynamic Immune Response Shapes COVID-19 Progression. *Cell Host Microbe* **2020**, *27*, 879–882.e2. [CrossRef] [PubMed]
25. Dimopoulos, G.; De Mast, Q.; Markou, N.; Theodorakopoulou, M.; Komnos, A.; Mouktaroudi, M.; Netea, M.G.; Spyridopoulos, T.; Verheggen, R.J.; Hoogerwerf, J.; et al. Favorable Anakinra Responses in Severe Covid-19 Patients with Secondary Hemophagocytic Lymphohistiocytosis. *Cell Host Microbe* **2020**. [CrossRef] [PubMed]
26. Day, J.W.; Fox, T.A.; Halsey, R.; Carpenter, B.; Kottaridis, P.D. IL-1 blockade with anakinra in acute leukaemia patients with severe COVID-19 pneumonia appears safe and may result in clinical improvement. *Br. J. Haematol.* **2020**. [CrossRef] [PubMed]
27. De Luca, A.; Smeekens, S.P.; Casagrande, A.; Iannitti, R.; Conway, K.L.; Gresnigt, M.; Begun, J.; Plantinga, T.; Joosten, L.A.B.; Van Der Meer, J.W.M.; et al. IL-1 receptor blockade restores autophagy and reduces inflammation in chronic granulomatous disease in mice and in humans. *Proc. Natl. Acad. Sci. USA* **2014**, *111*, 3526–3531. [CrossRef]
28. Iannitti, R.G.; Napolioni, V.; Oikonomou, V.; De Luca, A.; Galosi, C.; Pariano, M.; Massi-Benedetti, C.; Borghi, M.; Puccetti, M.; Lucidi, V.; et al. IL-1 receptor antagonist ameliorates inflammasome-dependent inflammation in murine and human cystic fibrosis. *Nat. Commun.* **2016**, *7*, 10791. [CrossRef]
29. Zhang, X.; Tan, Y.; Ling, Y.; Lu, G.; Liu, F.; Yi, Z.; Jia, X.; Wu, M.; Shi, B.; Xu, S.; et al. Viral and host factors related to the clinical outcome of COVID-19. *Nature* **2020**, 1–7. [CrossRef]
30. Liu, T.; Zhang, J.; Yang, Y.; Ma, H.; Li, Z.; Zhang, J.; Cheng, J.; Zhang, X.; Zhao, Y.; Xia, Z.; et al. The role of interleukin-6 in monitoring severe case of coronavirus disease 2019. *EMBO Mol. Med.* **2020**, e12421. [CrossRef]
31. Mazzoni, A.; Salvati, L.; Maggi, L.; Capone, M.; Vanni, A.; Spinicci, M.; Mencarini, J.; Caporale, R.; Peruzzi, B.; Antonelli, A.; et al. Impaired immune cell cytotoxicity in severe COVID-19 is IL-6 dependent. *J. Clin. Investig.* **2020**. [CrossRef]
32. Borger, P.; Koeter, G.H.; Timmerman, A.J.; Vellenga, A.; Tomee, J.F.; Kauffman, H.F. Protease from *Aspergillus fumigatus* induce interleukin (IL)-6 and IL-8 producin in airway epithelial cell lines by transcriptional mechanisms. *J. Infect. Dis.* **1999**, *180*, 1267–1274. [CrossRef] [PubMed]
33. Toniati, P.; Piva, S.; Cattalini, M.; Garrafa, E.; Regola, F.; Castelli, F.; Franceschini, F.; Airo, P.; Bazzani, C.; Research, B.I.; et al. Tocilizumab for the treatment of severe COVID-19 pneumonia with hyperinflammatory syndrome and acute respiratory failure: A single center study of 100 patients in brescia, Italy. *Autoimmun. Rev.* **2020**. [CrossRef] [PubMed]
34. Cenci, E.; Mencacci, A.; Casagrande, A.; Mosci, P.; Bistoni, F.; Romani, L. Impaired antifungal effector activity but not inflammatory cell recruitment in interleukin-6-deficient mice with invasive pulmonary aspergillosis. *J. Infect. Dis.* **2001**, *184*, 610–617. [CrossRef]
35. Huang, C.; Wang, Y.; Li, X.; Ren, L.; Zhao, J.; Hu, Y.; Zhang, L.; Fan, G.; Xu, J.; Cheng, Z.; et al. Clinical features of patients infected with 2019 novel coronavirus in Wuhan, China. *Lancet* **2020**, *395*, 497–506. [CrossRef]
36. Qin, C.; Zhou, L.; Hu, Z.; Zhang, S.; Yang, S.; Tao, Y.; Xie, C.; Ma, K.; Shang, K.; Wang, W.; et al. Dysregulation of Immune Response in Patients With Coronavirus 2019 (COVID-19) in Wuhan, China. *Clin. Infect. Dis.* **2020**. [CrossRef] [PubMed]
37. Giamarellos-Bourboulis, E.; Netea, M.G.; Rovina, N.; Akinosoglou, K.; Antoniadou, A.; Antonakos, N.; Damoraki, G.; Gkavogianni, T.; Adami, M.-E.; Katsaounou, P.; et al. Complex Immune Dysregulation in COVID-19 Patients with Severe Respiratory Failure. *Cell Host Microbe* **2020**, *27*, 992–1000.e3. [CrossRef]

38. Stanzani, M.; Vianelli, N.; Cavo, M.; Kontoyiannis, D.P.; Lewis, R.E. Development and internal validation of a model for predicting 60-day risk of invasive mould disease in patients with haematological malignancies. *J. Infect.* **2019**, *78*, 484–490. [CrossRef]
39. Netea, M.G.; Giamarellos-Bourboulis, E.J.; Dominguez-Andres, J.; Curtis, N.; Crevel, R.; Veerdonk, F.L.; Bonten, M. Trained immunity: A tool for reducing susceptibility to and the severity of SARS-CoV-2 infection. *Cell* **2020**, *181*, 969–977. [CrossRef]
40. Van De Veerdonk, F.L.; Kolwijck, E.; A Lestrade, P.P.; Hodiamont, C.J.; Rijnders, B.J.; Van Paassen, J.; Haas, P.-J.; Dos Santos, C.O.; Kampinga, G.; Bergmans, D.C.; et al. Influenza-associated Aspergillosis in Critically Ill Patients. *Am. J. Respir. Crit. Care Med.* **2017**, *196*, 524–527. [CrossRef]
41. Jenks, J.D.; Mehta, S.R.; Taplitz, R.; Aslam, S.; Reed, S.L.; Hoenigl, M. Point-of-care diagnosis of invasive aspergillosis in non-neutropenic patients: Aspergillus Galactomannan Lateral Flow Assay versus Aspergillus -specific Lateral Flow Device test in bronchoalveolar lavage. *Mycoses* **2019**, *62*, 230–236. [CrossRef] [PubMed]
42. Jenks, J.D.; Salzer, H.J.F.; Hoenigl, M. Improving the rates of Aspergillus detection: An update on current diagnostic strategies. *Expert Rev. Anti-infective Ther.* **2018**, *17*, 39–50. [CrossRef]
43. Donnelly, J.P.; Chen, S.C.; A Kauffman, C.; Steinbach, W.J.; Baddley, J.W.; Verweij, P.E.; Clancy, C.J.; Wingard, J.R.; Lockhart, S.R.; Groll, A.H.; et al. Revision and Update of the Consensus Definitions of Invasive Fungal Disease From the European Organization for Research and Treatment of Cancer and the Mycoses Study Group Education and Research Consortium. *Clin. Infect. Dis.* **2019**. [CrossRef] [PubMed]
44. Blot, S.; Taccone, F.S.; Abeele, A.-M.V.D.; Bulpa, P.; Meersseman, W.; Brusselaers, N.; Dimopoulos, G.; Paiva, J.A.; Misset, B.; Rello, J.; et al. A Clinical Algorithm to Diagnose Invasive Pulmonary Aspergillosis in Critically Ill Patients. *Am. J. Respir. Crit. Care Med.* **2012**, *186*, 56–64. [CrossRef] [PubMed]
45. Bassetti, M.; Giacobbe, D.R.; Grecchi, C.; Rebuffi, C.; Zuccaro, V.; Scudeller, L. Performance of existing definitions and tests for the diagnosis of invasive aspergillosis in critically ill, adult patients: A systematic review with qualitative evidence synthesis. *J. Infect.* **2020**, *81*, 131–146. [CrossRef]
46. Bassetti, M.; Scudeller, L.; Giacobbe, D.R.; Lamoth, F.; Righi, E.; Zuccaro, V.; Grecchi, C.; Rebuffi, C.; Akova, M.; Alastruey-Izquierdo, A.; et al. Developing definitions for invasive fungal diseases in critically ill adult patients in intensive care units. Protocol of the FUN gal infections Definitions in ICU patients (FUNDICU) project. *Mycoses* **2019**, *62*, 310–319. [CrossRef]
47. Arkel, A.L.E.; Rijpstra, T.A.; Belderbos, H.N.A.; Wijngaarden, P.; Verweij, P.E.; Bentvelsen, R.G. COVID-19 Associated pulmonary aspergillosis. *Am. J. Respir. Crit. Care Med.* **2020**. [CrossRef]
48. Russel, C.D.; Millar, J.E.; Baillie, J.K. Clinical evidence does not support corticosteroid treatment for 2019-nCoV lung injury. *Lancet* **2020**, *395*, 473–475. [CrossRef]
49. Cox, M.J.; Loman, N.; Bogaert, D.; Grady, J.O. Co-infections: Potentially lethal and unexplored in COVID-19. *Lancet Microbe* **2020**. [CrossRef]
50. Koehler, P.; Cornely, O.A.; Böttiger, B.W.; Dusse, F.; Eichenauer, D.A.; Fuchs, F.; Hallek, M.; Jung, N.; Klein, F.; Persigehl, T.; et al. COVID-19 associated pulmonary aspergillosis. *Mycoses* **2020**, *63*, 528–534. [CrossRef]
51. Alanio, A.; Dellière, S.; Fodil, S.; Bretagne, S.; Megarbane, B. Prevalence of putative invasive pulmonary aspergillosis in critically ill patients with COVID-19. *Lancet Respir. Med.* **2020**. [CrossRef]
52. Rutsaert, L.; Steinfort, N.; Hunsel, T.V.; Bomans, P.; Mertes, H.; Dits, H.; Regenmortel, N.V. COVID-19-associated invasive pulmonary aspergillosis. *Ann. Intensive Care* **2020**, *10*, 71. [CrossRef] [PubMed]
53. Spagnolo, P.; Balestro, E.; Aliberti, S.; Cocconcelli, E.; Biondini, D.; Casa, G.D.; Sverzellati, N.; Maher, T.M. Pulmonary fibrosis secondary to COVID-19: A call to arms? *Lancet Respir. Med.* **2020**. [CrossRef]
54. Chen, N.; Zhou, M.; Dong, X.; Qu, J.; Gong, F.; Han, Y.; Qiu, Y.; Wang, J.; Liu, Y.; Wei, Y.; et al. Epidemiological and Clinical Characteristics of 99 Cases of 2019-Novel Coronavirus (2019-nCoV) Pneumonia in Wuhan, China. *SSRN Electron. J.* **2020**, *395*, 507–513. [CrossRef]
55. Du, Y.; Tu, L.; Zhu, P.; Mu, M.; Wang, R.; Yang, P.; Wang, X.; Hu, C.; Ping, R.; Li, T.; et al. Clinical features of 85 fatal cases of COVID-19 from Wuhan: A retrospective observational study. *Am J. Respir. Crit. Care Med.* **2020**, *201*, 1372–1379. [CrossRef]
56. Wang, D.; Hu, B.; Hu, C.; Zhu, F.; Liu, X.; Zhang, J.; Wang, B.; Xiang, H.; Cheng, Z.; Xiong, Y.; et al. Clinical Characteristics of 138 Hospitalized Patients With 2019 Novel Coronavirus–Infected Pneumonia in Wuhan, China. *JAMA* **2020**, *323*, 1061. [CrossRef]

57. Blaize, M.; Mayaux, J.; Nabet, C.; Lampros, A.; Marcelin, A.G.; Thellier, M.; Piarroux, R.; Demoule, A.; Fekkar, A. Fatal invasive aspergillosis and coronavirus disease in an immunocompetent patient. *Emerg. Infect. Dis.* **2020**, 26. [CrossRef]
58. Lescure, F.X.; Bouadma, L.; Nguyen, D.; Parisey, M.; Wicky, P.H.; Behillil, S.; Gaymard, A.; Bouscambert-Duchamp, M.; Donati, F.; Le Hingrat, Q.; et al. Clinical and virological data of the first cases of COVID-19 in Europe: A case series. *Lancet. Infect. Dis.* **2020**. [CrossRef]
59. Antinori, S.; Rech, R.; Galimberti, L.; Castelli, A.; Angeli, E.; Fossali, T.; Bernasconi, D.; Covizzi, A.; Bonazzetti, C.; Torre, A.; et al. Invasive pulmonary aspergillosis complicating SARS-CoV-2 pneumonia: A diagnostic challenge. *Travel Med. Infect. Dis.* **2020**, 101752. [CrossRef]
60. Prattes, J.; Valentin, T.; Hoenigl, M.; Talakic, E.; Alexander, C.R.; Eller, P. Invasive pulmonary aspergillosis complicating COVID-19 in the ICU—A case. *Med. Mycol. Case Rep.* **2020**. [CrossRef]
61. Lahmer, T.; Rasch, S.; Spinner, C.; Geisler, F.; Schmid, R.M.; Huber, W. Invasive pulmonary aspergillosis in severe COVID-19 pneumonia. *Clin. Microbiol. Infect.* **2020**. [CrossRef]
62. Meijer, E.F.J.; Dofferhoff, A.S.M.; Hoiting, O.; Buil, J.B.; Meis, J.F. Azole resistant COVID-19 associated pulmonary aspergillosis in an immunocompetent host: A case report. *J. Fungi* **2020**, *2*, 79. [CrossRef] [PubMed]
63. Sharma, A.; Hofmeyr, A.; Bansal, A.; Thakkar, D.; Lam, L.; Harrington, Z.; Bhonagiri, D. COVID-19 associated pulmonary aspergillosis (CAPA): An Australian case report. *Med Mycol. Case Rep.* **2020**. [CrossRef]
64. Cornely, O.A.; Hoenigl, M.; Lass-Flörl, C.; Chen, S.; Kontoyiannis, D.P.; Morrissey, C.O.; Thmpson, G.R. Mycoses Study Group Education and Research Consortium (MSG-ERC) and the European Confederation of Medical Mycology (ECMM). Defining breakthrough invasive fungal infection-position paper of the mycoses study group education and research consortium and the european confederation of medical mycology. *Mycoses* **2019**, *62*, 716–729. [PubMed]
65. Clark, C.; Drummond, R.A. The hidden cost of modern medical interventions: How medical advances have shaped the prevalence of human fungal disease. *Pathogens* **2019**, *8*, 45. [CrossRef] [PubMed]
66. Sanguinetti, M.; Posteraro, B.; Beigelman-aubry, C.; Lamoth, F.; Dunet, V.; Slavin, M.; Richardson, M.D. Diagnosis and treatment of invasive fungal infections: Looking ahead. *J. Antimicrob. Chemother.* **2019**, *74*, ii27–ii37. [CrossRef] [PubMed]
67. Critchley, J.A.; Carey, I.M.; Harris, T.; DeWilde, S.; Hosking, F.J.; Cook, D.G. Glycemic control and risk of infections among people with type 1 or type 2 diabetes in a large primary care cohort study. *Diabetes Care* **2018**, *41*, 2127–2135. [CrossRef]
68. Danesh, J.; Collins, R.; Peto, R. Chronic infections and coronary heart disease: Is there a link? *Lancet* **1997**, *350*, 430–436. [CrossRef]
69. Hotez, P.J. Linking tropical infections to hypertension: New comorbid disease. *J. Am. Heart. Assoc.* **2019**, *8*, e03984. [CrossRef]
70. Ader, F.; Nseir, S.; Berre, R.L.; Leroy, S.; Tillie-Leblond, I.; Marquette, C.H.; Durocher, A. Invasive pulmonary *aspergillosis* in chronic obstructive pulmonary disease: An emerging fungal pathogen. *Clin. Microbiol. Infect.* **2005**, *11*, 427–429. [CrossRef]
71. Wang, J.; Yang, Q.; Zhang, P.; Sheng, J.; Zhou, J.; Qu, T. Clinical characteristics of invasive pulmonary aspergillosis in patients with COVID-19 in Zhejiang, China: A retrospective case series. *Crit Care* **2020**, *24*, 299. [CrossRef] [PubMed]
72. Zhang, G.; Hu, C.; Luo, L.; Fang, F.; Chen, Y.; Li, J.; Peng, Z.; Pan, H. Clinical features and short-term outcomes of 221 patients with COVID-19 in Wuhan, China. *J. Clin. Virol.* **2020**, *127*, 104364. [CrossRef] [PubMed]
73. Arastehfar, A.; Wickes, B.L.; Ilkit, M.; Pincus, D.H.; Daneshnia, F.; Pan, W.; Fang, W.; Boekhout, T. Identification of mycoses in developing countries. *J. Fungi* **2019**, *5*, 90. [CrossRef] [PubMed]
74. Eigl, S.; Spiess, B.; Heldt, S.; Rabensteiner, J.; Prüller, F.; Flick, H.; Boch, T.; Hoenigl, M.; Prattes, J.; Neumeister, P.; et al. Galactomannan testing and Aspergillus PCR in same-day bronchoalveolar lavage and blood samples for diagnosis of invasive aspergillosis. *Med. Mycol.* **2016**, *55*, 528–534. [CrossRef]
75. Chindamporn, A.; Chakrabarti, A.; Li, R.; Sun, P.-L.; Tan, B.-H.; Chua, M.; Wahyuningsih, R.; Patel, A.; Liu, Z.; Chen, Y.-C.; et al. Survey of laboratory practices for diagnosis of fungal infection in seven Asian countries: An Asia Fungal Working Group (AFWG) initiative. *Med. Mycol.* **2017**, *56*, 416–425. [CrossRef] [PubMed]

76. Kalil, A.C.; Thomas, P.G. Influenza virus-related critical illness: Pathophysiology and epidemiology. *Crit. Care* **2019**, *23*, 258. [CrossRef]
77. Lestrade, P.P.A.; Meis, J.F.; Melchers, W.J.G.; Verweij, P.E. Triazole resistance in *Aspergillus fumigatus*: Recent insights and challenges for patient management. *Clin. Microbiol. Infect.* **2019**, *25*, 799–806. [CrossRef]
78. Wahidi, M.M.; Lamb, C.; Murgu, S.; Musani, A.; Shojaee, S.; Sachdeva, A.; Maldonado, F.; Mahmood, K.; Kinsey, M.; Sethi, S.; et al. American Association for Bronchology and Interventional Pulmonology (AABIP) Statement on the Use of Bronchoscopy and Respiratory Specimen Collection in Patients with Suspected or Confirmed COVID-19 Infection. *J. Bronchol. Interv. Pulmonol.* **2020**. [CrossRef]
79. Patterson, T.F.; Thompson, G.R., III; Denning, D.W.; Fishman, J.A.; Hadley, S.; Herbrecht, R.; Kontoyiannis, D.P.; Marr, K.A.; Morrison, V.A.; Segal, B.H.; et al. Practice guidelines for the diagnosis and management of aspergillosis: 2016 update by the infectious diseases society of america. *Clin. Infect. Dis.* **2016**, *63*, e1–e60. [CrossRef]
80. Ullmann, A.; Aguado, J.; Arikan-Akdagli, S.; Denning, D.; Groll, A.; Lagrou, K.; Lass-Flörl, C.; Lewis, R.; Munoz, P.; E Verweij, P.; et al. Diagnosis and management of Aspergillus diseases: Executive summary of the 2017 ESCMID-ECMM-ERS guideline. *Clin. Microbiol. Infect.* **2018**, *24*, e1–e38. [CrossRef]
81. Hoenigl, M.; Duettmann, W.; Raggam, R.B.; Seeber, K.; Troppan, K.; Fruhwald, S.; Prüller, F.; Wagner, J.; Valentin, T.; Zollner-Schwetz, I.; et al. Potential Factors for Inadequate Voriconazole Plasma Concentrations in Intensive Care Unit Patients and Patients with Hematological Malignancies. *Antimicrob. Agents Chemother.* **2013**, *57*, 3262–3267. [CrossRef] [PubMed]
82. Jenks, J.D.; Mehta, S.R.; Hoenigl, M. Broad spectrum triazoles for invasive mould infections in adults: Which drug and when? *Med. Mycol.* **2019**, *57*, S168–S178. [CrossRef] [PubMed]
83. Baniasadi, S.; Farzanegan, B.; Alehashem, M. Important drug classes associated with potential drug – drug interactions in critically ill patients: Highlights for cardiothoracic intensivists. *Ann. Intensive Care* **2015**, *5*, 10–14. [CrossRef] [PubMed]
84. McCreary, E.K.; Pogue, J.M. Coronavirus Disease 2019 Treatment: A Review of early and emerging options. *Open. Forum. Infect Dis.* **2020**, *7*, ofaa105. [CrossRef]
85. Jenks, J.D.; Salzer, H.J.F.; Prattes, J.; Krause, R.; Buchheidt, D.; Hoenigl, M. Spotlight on isavuconazole in the treatment of invasive aspergillosis and mucormycosis: Design, development, and place in therapy. *Drug. Des. Devel. Ther.* **2018**, *12*, 1033–1044. [CrossRef]
86. Hoenigl, M.; Prattes, J.; Neumeister, P.; Wölfler, A.; Krause, R. Real- world challenges and unmet needs in the diagnosis and treatment of suspected invasive pulmonary aspergillosis in patients with haematological diseases: An illustrative case study. *Mycoses* **2018**, *61*, 201–205. [CrossRef]
87. Puelles, V.G.; Lütgehetmann, M.; Lindenmeyer, M.T.; Sperhake, J.P.; Wong, M.N.; Allweiss, L.; Chilla, S.; Heinemann, A.; Wanner, N.; Liu, S.; et al. Multiorgan and Renal Tropism of SARS-CoV-2. *N. Engl. J. Med.* **2020**. [CrossRef]
88. Takano, T.; Akiyama, M.; Doki, T.; Hohdatsu, T. Antiviral activity of itraconazole against type I feline coronavirus infection. *Vet Res.* **2019**, *50*, 5. [CrossRef]
89. Nield, B.; Larsen, S.R.; van Hal, S.J. Clinical experience with new formulation SUBA(R)-itraconazole for prophylaxis in patients undergoing stem cell transplantation or treatment for haematological malignancies. *J. Antimicrob. Chemother.* **2019**, *74*, 3049–3055. [CrossRef]
90. Aruanno, M.; Glampedakis, E.; Lamoth, F. Echinocandins for the Treatment of Invasive Aspergillosis: From Laboratory to Bedside. *Antimicrob. Agents Chemother.* **2019**, *63*, e00399-19. [CrossRef]
91. Kupferschmidt, K. New drugs target growing threat of fatal fungi. *Science* **2019**, *366*, 407. [CrossRef]
92. Wiederhold, N.P.; Locke, J.B.; Daruwala, P.; Bartizal, K. Rezafungin (CD101) demonstrates potent in vitro activity against *Aspergillus*, including azole-resistant *Aspergillus fumigatus* isolates and cryptic species. *J. Antimicrob. Chemother.* **2018**, *73*, 3063–3067. [CrossRef]
93. Cevik, M.; Bamford, C.G.G.; Ho, A. COVID-19 pandemic-a focused review for clinicians. *Clin. Microbiol. Infect.* **2020**. [CrossRef]
94. Rijnders, B.L.; Schauwvlieghe, A.F.A.D.; Wauters, J. Influenza-Associated Pulmonary Aspergillosis: A Local or Global Lethal Combination? *Clin. Infect. Dis.* **2020**. [CrossRef] [PubMed]
95. Ackermann, M.; Verleden, S.E.; Kuehnel, M.; Haverich, A.; Welte, T.; Laenger, F.; Vanstapel, A.; Werlein, C.; Stark, H.; Tzankov, A.; et al. Pulmonary Vascular Endothelialitis, Thrombosis, and Angiogenesis in Covid-19. *N. Engl. J. Med.* **2020**. [CrossRef] [PubMed]

96. Thompson, G.R., III; Cornely, O.A.; Pappas, P.G.; Patterson, T.F.; Hoenigl, M.; Jenks, J.D.; Clancy, C.J.; Nguyen, M.H.; Mycoses Study Group (MSG) and European Confederation of Medical Mycology (ECMM). Invasive Aspergillosis as an Underrecognized Superinfection in COVID-19. *Open Forum Infect. Dis.* **2020**. [CrossRef]
97. Verweij, P.E.; Gangneux, J.-P.; Bassetti, M.; Brüggemann, R.J.M.; A Cornely, O.; Koehler, P.; Lass-Flörl, C.; Van De Veerdonk, F.L.; Chakrabarti, A.; Hoenigl, M. Diagnosing COVID-19-associated pulmonary aspergillosis. *Lancet Microbe* **2020**, *1*, e53–e55. [CrossRef]

Journal of *Fungi*

MDPI

Article

Is the COVID-19 Pandemic a Good Time to Include *Aspergillus* Molecular Detection to Categorize Aspergillosis in ICU Patients? A Monocentric Experience

Jean-Pierre Gangneux [1,2,*], Florian Reizine [3], Hélène Guegan [1,2], Kieran Pinceaux [3], Pierre Le Balch [3], Emilie Prat [1], Romain Pelletier [1], Sorya Belaz [1], Mathieu Le Souhaitier [3], Yves Le Tulzo [3], Philippe Seguin [4], Mathieu Lederlin [5], Jean-Marc Tadié [3] and Florence Robert-Gangneux [1,2]

1 Service de Parasitologie-Mycologie, CHU Rennes, F-35033 Rennes, France; helene.guegan@chu-rennes.fr (H.G.); emilie.prat@chu-rennes.fr (E.P.); romain.pelletier@chu-rennes.fr (R.P.); sorya.belaz@chu-rennes.fr (S.B.); florence.robert-gangneux@univ-rennes1.fr (F.R.-G.)
2 Irset (Institut de Recherche en Santé, Environnement et Travail)–UMR_S 1085, Univ Rennes, CHU Rennes, Inserm, EHESP, F-35000 Rennes, France
3 Maladies Infectieuses et Réanimation Médicale, CHU Rennes, F-35033 Rennes, France; florian.reizine@chu-rennes.fr (F.R.); kieran.pinceaux@chu-rennes.fr (K.P.); pierre.le.balch@chu-rennes.fr (P.L.B.); mathieu.lesouhaitier@chu-rennes.fr (M.L.S.); yves.le.tulzo@chu-rennes.fr (Y.L.T.); jeanmarc.tadie@chu-rennes.fr (J.-M.T.)
4 Service de Réanimation Chirurgicale, CHU Rennes, F-35033 Rennes, France; philippe.seguin@chu-rennes.fr
5 Service d'Imagerie Médicale, CHU Rennes, F-35033 Rennes, France; mathieu.lederlin@chu-rennes.fr
* Correspondence: Jean-pierre.gangneux@univ-rennes1.fr

Received: 12 June 2020; Accepted: 6 July 2020; Published: 10 July 2020

Abstract: (1) Background: The diagnosis of invasive aspergillosis (IA) in an intensive care unit (ICU) remains a challenge and the COVID-19 epidemic makes it even harder. Here, we evaluated *Aspergillus* PCR input to help classifying IA in SARS-CoV-2-infected patients. (2) Methods: 45 COVID-19 patients were prospectively monitored twice weekly for *Aspergillus* markers and anti-*Aspergillus* serology. We evaluated the concordance between (I) *Aspergillus* PCR and culture in respiratory samples, and (II) blood PCR and serum galactomannan. Patients were classified as putative/proven/colonized using AspICU algorithm and two other methods. (3) Results: The concordance of techniques applied on respiratory and blood samples was moderate (kappa = 0.58 and kappa = 0.63, respectively), with a higher sensitivity of PCR. According to AspICU, 9/45 patients were classified as putative IA. When incorporating PCR results, 15 were putative IA because they met all criteria, probably with a lack of specificity in the context of COVID-19. Using a modified AspICU algorithm, eight patients were classified as colonized and seven as putative IA. (4) Conclusion: An appreciation of the fungal burden using PCR and *Aspergillus* serology was added to propose a modified AspICU algorithm. This proof of concept seemed relevant, as it was in agreement with the outcome of patients, but will need validation in larger cohorts.

Keywords: invasive aspergillosis; putative; probable; COVID-19; Sars-CoV-2; ICU; PCR; *Aspergillus*; galactomannan; classification

1. Introduction

Molecular tools as diagnostic criteria for invasive fungal diseases (IFD) has long been questioned because of a lack of reproducibility and insufficient standardization of protocols. Thanks to initiatives such as FPCRI (www.fpcri.eu [1]) and to the dramatic improvement of the quality assessment of molecular technics, *Aspergillus* PCR is now included in the new EORTC criteria for classification [2]. Regarding intensive care units (ICU) patients, the classification of IFD mainly refers on criteria adapted from neutropenic patients or relies on single center experiences. One algorithm has emerged as a valuable tool to classify invasive aspergillosis (IA) in ICU patients: the AspICU algorithm [3]. This classification is considered as robust because it has been evaluated in patients for whom autopsy results were available, but it is quite awkward to use in routine practice, particularly in COVID-19 patients with clinical and CT-scan signs hard to interpret [4]. Besides, it does not include molecular markers, which are now used routinely [5].

During COVID-19, patients presenting an acute respiratory distress syndrome (ARDS) shared risk factors and underlying diseases classically reported for IA, such as intubation and mechanical ventilation, corticosteroid therapy, immunological storm with high production of inflammatory cytokines. Warnings following preliminary cohort studies from various countries prompted the monitoring of fungal colonization and co-infections in SARS-CoV-2-infected patients hospitalized in an ICU. However, the entry criterion for putative IA, according to Blot et al., is an *Aspergillus*-positive culture endotracheal aspirate, which may lack specificity. In the recent review by Arastehfar et al. [6], many COVID-19-associated pulmonary aspergillosis (CAPA) benefited from galactomannan (GM) testing of bronchoalveolar fluid (BALF) or even of tracheal aspirates (not approved by the manufacturer). However, some laboratories, such as ours, have stopped various manipulations of highly SARS-CoV-2-infected samples in order to limit the exposure of laboratory technicians to viral infection. Then, direct examination of respiratory samples or galactomannan (GM) determination in broncho-alveolar lavage have thus been replaced by the systematic use of molecular tools. While performances of blood biomarkers such as GM, (1-3)β-D-glucan (BDG) or *Aspergillus* DNA detection are well evaluated in neutropenic patients, their clinical value is far less known in other conditions and still need evaluation in an ICU.

Here, our objective was to evaluate the concordance between molecular detection of *Aspergillus* in respiratory and culture and concordance between blood PCR and serum GM. We also aimed at assessing the ability of *Aspergillus* PCRs to help categorizing patients in the continuum of colonization to invasive infection in COVID-19 patients. Arguments to complement AspICU criteria are suggested.

2. Materials and Methods

2.1. Population of Patients

Forty-five intubated and mechanically ventilated patients hospitalized in a "COVID-19 ICU" of Rennes teaching hospital were screened for this study and benefited from a systematic monitoring to detect *Aspergillus*.

The hospital's ethics committee (N 20-56 obtained the 30 April 2020) approved the study. The presence of SARS-CoV-2 in respiratory specimens (nasal and pharyngeal swabs or sputum) was detected by real time reverse transcription-polymerase chain reaction (RT-PCR) methods.

The following data were recorded: age, patient's preexisting condition (current smoking, diabetes, hypertension, cardiovascular disease, pulmonary disease, and kidney disease), body mass index, ICU length of stay, duration of mechanical ventilation, ventilator-free days at day 28, need for prone position ventilation, and death in the ICU. Initial clinical laboratory workup included a complete blood count and serum biochemical tests. Chest CT scans were performed during the ICU hospitalization. The Simplified Acute Physiology Score (SAPS II) and the Sepsis-Related Organ Failure Assessment (SOFA) score at admission in ICU, at day 7 and 14 days after admission were used to assess severity [7,8].

2.2. *Aspergillus* Detection

Respiratory samples, either bronchial or endotracheal aspirates or bronchoalveolar lavages, were systematic twice weekly and *Aspergillus* detection was performed using culture and real-time quantitative PCR, but GM was not performed to avoid any risk of lab contamination.

Briefly, respiratory samples were first digested using *v/v* digestEUR (Eurobio) for 30 min under shaking. Mycological culture were performed after centrifugation of fluidified samples by inoculation of 100–200 μL of pellet on Sabouraud-Chloramphenicol dextrose Agar plates, and incubated for 7 days at 30 °C and 37 °C. Mold identification at genus or species complex level was performed microscopically, and confirmed at species level using MALDI-ToF mass spectrometry (MALDI Biotyper, Bruker France, Marne-la-Vallée, France), after fungal material extraction [9]. Spectrum profiles were then submitted to the Mass Spectrometry Identification (MSI) online database for definitive identification (https://msi.happy-dev.fr/ [10]).

For molecular detection, 200 μL of plain fluidified respiratory sample underwent immediate SARS-CoV-2 inactivation by heating at 56 °C overnight in ATL Lysis buffer (Qiagen, Saint-Quentin Fallavier, France), before DNA extraction using the EZ1 DSP virus kit (Qiagen) on a EZ1 Advanced XL device (Qiagen). Molecular detection of *A. fumigatus* was done using a 28S rDNA *Aspergillus*-targeted PCR, as previously published [11,12].

In case of *Aspergillus* positive culture and/or positive PCR in respiratory samples, additional tests were performed on serum, i.e., detection of GM (Platelia GM *Aspergillus*, Biorad, Marnes-la-Coquette, France), *Aspergillus* PCR and detection of anti-*Aspergillus* antibody by ELISA (Platelia IgG *Aspergillus*, Biorad) and in-house immunoelectrophoresis. Briefly, *Aspergillus* PCR was performed on 1 mL of serum extracted using MagNA Pure 24 Total NA Isolation kit (Roche diagnostics, Meylan, France) on a MagNA Pure 24 device (Roche diagnostics), according to manufacturer recommendations. DNA was eluted in a volume of 50 μL.

2.3. *Statistical Analysis*

Continuous variables were expressed as median (interquartile range, IQR) and compared using the nonparametric Mann–Whitney *U* or Kruskal–Wallis test. Dunn's correction tests were performed if multiple comparisons were requested. Qualitative data were compared using Chi-square test. Tests were two-sided with significance set at α less than 0.05.

Concordance between categorical results from diagnostic tests was performed using the percent agreement coefficient and Cohen's kappa coefficient (κ). When comparing quantitative data, an ANOVA test was performed. All data were analyzed with GraphPad Prism 8.4 (GraphPad Software, La Jolla, CA, USA).

3. Results

3.1. *Patient Aspergillus Status*

A cohort of 45 COVID-19 intubated and mechanically ventilated patients for ARDS was followed. Patients benefited from a systematic screening for *Aspergillus.* Overall, 211 respiratory samples (culture and PCR) and 32 serum samples (GM detection and *Aspergillus* PCR) were collected. The mean number of respiratory samples until patient discharge from ICU was 3.8 (median = 3).

We categorized these 45 patients according to the AspICU algorithm and propose two alternative classification methods presented in Table 1: the AspICU algorithm associated to PCR results in respiratory and serum samples, and a modified AspICU proposal. Thirty patients did not present any biological criteria of aspergillosis with any of the algorithms. According to the AspICU classification incorporating PCR detection, 15 were classified as having putative aspergillosis because they met all criteria reported by Blot et al., i.e., compatible clinical signs, abnormal thoracic medical imaging on CT scan and positive screening for *Aspergillus* on respiratory samples. However, in this particular context of COVID-19 with all ARDS patients presenting compatible clinical signs and abnormal chest

CT imaging in all likelihood lacking specificity, we decided to use a modified AspICU algorithm taking into account blood markers; we classified eight patients as colonized and seven patients with a putative/probable IA (Tables 1 and 2).

Table 1. Diagnostic criteria of the AspICU clinical algorithm according to Blot et al., 2012, and proposal of a modified AspICU algorithm.

Classification	AspICU According to Blot et al., 2012 [3]	AspICU Algorithm Incorporating PCR	Modified AspICU Algorithm Incorporating PCR, Serology and Angioinvasion Biomarkers
Definition of colonization	*Aspergillus*-positive culture endotracheal aspirate alone	*Aspergillus*-positive culture/PCR endotracheal aspirate alone	*Aspergillus*-positive culture/PCR endotracheal aspirate in one sample, not confirmed on a second sample or using blood biomarker
Definition of putative IA	>1 criterion among: 1. *Aspergillus*-positive culture endotracheal aspirate 2. Compatible clinical signs 3. Abnormal thoracic medical imaging on CT scan or X-ray 4a. Host risk factors Or 4b. Semiquantitative *Aspergillus*-positive culture of BAL fluid + positive direct microscopy	>1 criterion among: 1. *Aspergillus*-positive culture/PCR endotracheal aspirate 2. Compatible clinical signs 3. Abnormal thoracic medical imaging on CT scan or X-ray 4a. Host risk factors Or 4b. Semiquantitative *Aspergillus*-positive culture/PCR of BAL fluid + positive direct microscopy	>1 criterion among: 1. *Aspergillus*-positive culture/PCR endotracheal aspirate in repeated samples with negative anti-*Aspergillus* antibody testing 2. Compatible clinical signs 3. Abnormal thoracic medical imaging on CT scan or X-ray 4a. Host risk factors Or 4b. Semiquantitative *Aspergillus*-positive culture/PCR of BAL fluid + positive direct microscopy
Definition of probable IA	-	-	Putative IA + one positive blood biomarker (GM and/or PCR)
Definition of proven IA	Positive histopathology	Positive histopathology	Positive histopathology

GM: galactomannan.

Table 2. Classification of 45 COVID-19 patients with ARDS according to AspICU and to modified AspICU algorithms.

Classification	AspICU According to Blot et al., 2012 [3]	AspICU Algorithm Incorporating PCR	Modified AspICU Algorithm Incorporating PCR, Serology and Angioinvasion Biomarkers
No infection	36	30	30
Colonization	0	0	8
Putative IA	9	15	4
Probable IA	-	-	3
Proven IA	0	0	0

3.2. Demographic, Clinical and Biological Characteristics

Demographic, clinical and biological baseline characteristics at admission are detailed in Table 3 and Table S1. Basic demographic characteristics were well-balanced between the three groups of patients (no aspergillosis, *Aspergillus* colonization, putative/probable aspergillosis). Of note, we observed a high proportion (71.1%) of male patients in the study population. Clinical and biological baseline data did not differ among the three groups, except C-reactive protein which was higher in the "no aspergillosis" group. Regarding the severity scores at admission, no differences were observed either, among the groups of patients, but SAPS II and SOFA scores at day one tended to be higher in patients with putative invasive aspergillosis.

Table 3. Demographic characteristics and clinical and biological baseline characteristics.

Demographic Characteristics	All Patients (n = 45)	No Aspergillosis (n = 30)	*Aspergillus* Colonization (n = 8)	Putative/Probable Invasive Aspergillosis (n = 7)	p Value
Age, years	60 (53–71)	59 (54–68)	53 (51–71)	70 (63–75)	0.14
Sex Men Women	32 (71.1) 13 (28.9)	21 (70) 9 (30)	7 (87.5) 1 (12.5)	4 (57.1) 3 (42.8)	0.42
BMI	27 (24.4–31.4)	27.5 (24.7–32.3)	27 (25.2–30.7)	25.2 (23.2–26.4)	0.99
Current smoking	3 (6.7)	2 (4.4)	0	1 (12.5)	0.54
		Coexisting conditions			
Any	31 (68.9)	19 (63)	6 (75)	6 (85.7)	0.47
Diabetes	17 (37.8)	12 (40)	3 (37.5)	2 (28.6)	0.74
Hypertension	15 (33.3)	7 (23.3)	5 (62.5)	3 (42.9)	0.1
Solid cancer	1 (2.2)	1 (3.3)	0	0	0.77
Hemopathy	2 (4.4)	1 (3.3)	0	1 (14.3)	0.54
Cardiovascular disease	3 (6.7)	3 (10)	2 (25)	2 (28.6)	0.34
Chronic obstructive pulmonary disease	0	0	0	0	-
Chronic kidney disease	4 (8.9)	2 (6.7)	1 (12.5)	1 (14.3)	0.83
Temperature (°C)	38 (37–38.9)	37.5 (337–38.4)	38.2 (37.9–39)	38.2 (37.7–38.8)	0.29
Heart rate (/min)	100 (80–110)	94 (80–110)	104 (100–110)	102 (85–119)	0.63
Systolic pressure	94 (87–107)	93 (85–105)	103 (100–109)	90 (82–102)	0.34
White blood cell count (10^9/L)	9.8 (6.8–12.9)	9.7 (6.9–13)	9.9 (7–10.7)	9.9 (6.7–12.9)	0.97
Neutrophil count (10^9/L)	7.9 (4.5–10.8)	7 (4.9–10.5)	8.5 (5.2–8.6)	5.6 (3.5–10.4)	0.8
Lymphocyte count (10^9/L)	0.81 (0.58–1.11)	0.83 (0.53–1.14)	0.7 (0.63–1.1)	0.72 (0.58–0.81)	0.87
Hemoglobin (g/L)	10.8 (9.5–12.5)	10 (9.4–12)	11.8 (10.6–13.6)	11 (10.5–13.6)	0.12
Platelet count (10^9/L)	264 (194–357)	282 (220–364)	244 (184–347)	162 (129–262)	0.12
Total bilirubin concentration (μmol/L)	8 (5.5–12)	8.5 (6–12)	11 (9–13)	7 (5.5–8)	0.72
Creatinine (μmol/L)	81 (53–162)	71 (51–109)	81 (73–173)	101 (82–184)	0.15
C-reactive protein (CRP) (mg/L)	157 (112–263)	155 (112–265)	112 (102–131)	112 (109–178)	0.03
Ratio of PaO_2 to F_iO_2	152 (100–181)	164 (107–214)	120 (94–214)	136 (72–155)	0.25
SAPS II score on day 1	42 (31–57)	35 (30–58)	42 (21–55)	43 (35–82)	0.55
SOFA score on day 1	7 (2–11)	7 (4–10)	5 (2–10)	9 (2–12)	0.76

Data are presented as median (IQR: interquartiles), n (%). P values comparing *Aspergillus* colonization, invasive aspergillosis and no aspergillosis groups are tested by Kruskal–Wallis (continuous variables) or Chi-square test (categorical variables). Abbreviations: BMI: Body mass index; SAPS II: Simplified Acute Physiology Score II; SOFA: Sequential Organ Failure Assessment, PaO_2: arterial oxygen tension.

3.3. Concordance of Diagnostic Tools

Table 4 gathers the results of the techniques used for *Aspergillus* detection. DNA detection by PCR showed the highest sensitivity, with a number of positive respiratory samples near twice higher, compared to the culture. Only one sample grew in culture, whereas PCR was negative, but the species obtained in culture was *A. tubingensis* (*Nigri* complex species), which is theoretically not amplified when using the 28S-targeted PCR specific for *A. fumigatus*. Interestingly, the correlation between cultural and molecular quantification showed a significant difference between the two techniques, with a mean Cq threshold of 32.6 ± 0.7 when cultures were negative, highlighting the higher sensitivity of PCR (Figure 1).

Table 4. Concordance of PCR and cultures on respiratory samples (n = 211) to detect the presence of *Aspergillus*.

Respiratory Samples	Positive Culture	Negative Culture	Total
Positive PCR	15	19	34
Negative PCR	1 *	176	177
Total	16	191	211

* positive culture with *Aspergillus tubingensis* (*Nigri* section).

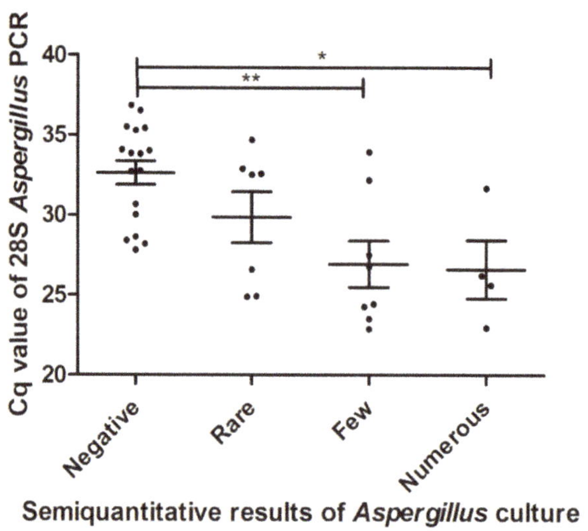

Figure 1. Correlation between molecular and cultural quantification of *Aspergillus* burden in respiratory samples (rare: 1–2 CFU/plate; few: 2–5; numerous: >5). * significantly different with $p < 0.05$. ** significantly different with $p < 0.01$.

Overall, the concordance coefficient between PCR and culture on respiratory samples was 90.52% with a Cohen's Kappa coefficient of 0.588. Regarding blood samples, three patients had a positive detection of a systemic biomarker: 3/3 had a positive PCR and 2/3 had a positive GM (Table 5). All three patients had a simultaneous detection of *Aspergillus* in respiratory samples by culture (n = 2) and/or PCR (n = 3). Overall, the concordance coefficient between PCR and culture on respiratory samples was 93.75% with a Cohen's Kappa coefficient of 0.632.

Table 5. Concordance of 28S PCR and galactomannan (GM) in serum samples (n = 32).

Serum Samples	Positive GM	Negative GM	Total
Positive PCR	2	1	3
Negative PCR	1	28	29
Total	3	29	32

3.4. Relevance of Various Tests and Categorization of Patients and Outcome

Table 6 presents the classification of the 45 patients using original or modified AspICU algorithms. It appears that using an AspICU algorithm, nine patients were considered as having a putative IA (22% of the cohort). When including PCR, the number of patients with putative IA would increase from 9 to 15 (33%) patients, while most patients might be only colonized because all presented compatible clinical signs and abnormal chest CT scan (Table 5). Regarding *Aspergillus* detection, eight patients had a single detection of fungi using culture and/or PCR in respiratory samples and thus were classified as colonized. One of these patients had a concomitant GM detection in serum (index = 0.551), was not treated and is still alive, thus was considered as a false positive result. Finally, seven (16%) patients presented a heavy burden of *Aspergillus* in the respiratory tract with repeated positive cultures and/or PCR. In order to rule out a chronic colonization before the episode, an anti-*Aspergillus* antibody testing was performed and showed negative results. These patients were classified as putative IA, and three of them could even be considered as probable IA because of a positive biomarker of angioinvasion (serum PCR and/or GM) in agreement with EORTC/MSG classification.

Table 6. Mycological results and classification of 45 COVID-19 patients with ARDS.

Patient	Respiratory Samples		Serum Samples		IA Classification According to		
	Aspergillus Positive Culture (nb Samples)	Positive 28S PCR (nb Samples)	GM Index > 0.5 (nb Samples)	Positive 28S PCR (nb Samples)	AspICU (Blot et al., 2012)	AspICU + PCR	Modified AspICU
1	5	5	2	2	putative	putative	probable
2	2	2	1	1	putative	putative	probable
3	0	3	0	1	no infection	putative	probable
4	4	6	0	0	putative	putative	putative
5	4	4	0	0	putative	putative	putative
6	2	5	0	0	putative	putative	putative
7	1	5	0	0	putative	putative	putative
8	1	1	0	0	putative	putative	colonization
9	1	0	1	0	putative	putative	colonization
10	1 *	0	0	0	putative	putative	colonization
11	0	1	0	0	no infection	putative	colonization
12	0	1	0	0	no infection	putative	colonization
13	0	1	0	0	no infection	putative	colonization
14	0	1	0	0	no infection	putative	colonization
15	0	1	0	0	no infection	putative	colonization
16–45	0	0	0	0	no infection	no infection	no infection
Total					9 putative (22%) 36 no infection	15 putative (33%) 30 no infection	3 probable (7%) 4 putative (9%) 8 colonizations (18%) 30 no infection

IA. Invasive aspergillosis, 1 * *Aspergillus tubingensis* (*Nigri* section).

Interestingly, following these classification criteria, CT scan abnormalities showed a gradation according to patient group. Diffuse reticular or alveolar opacities were observed in patients classified as probable IA (Figure 2), nodules in half of putative IA, and in colonized patients, only non-specific and hard to interpret signs in the context of COVID-19 infection could be described.

In addition, putative/probable aspergillosis patients appeared more severely ill than patients without aspergillosis, since SOFA score at day seven was significantly higher in this group ($p = 0.01$) with a continuum between no infection, colonization and IA (Table 5). Similarly, the mean ICU length of stay increased significantly from 12 days in patients without aspergillosis to 23 days in colonized patients, and 27 days in putative/probable invasive aspergillosis ($p = 0.02$). All patients with a putative/probable IA were treated either with voriconazole or isavuconazole. Only one colonized patient was treated with voriconazole. Six patients died; there was a trend towards higher mortality in the group of putative/probable IA compared to uninfected patients, although not significant (2/7; 28.6%) versus 4/30 (13.3%), respectively (Table 7).

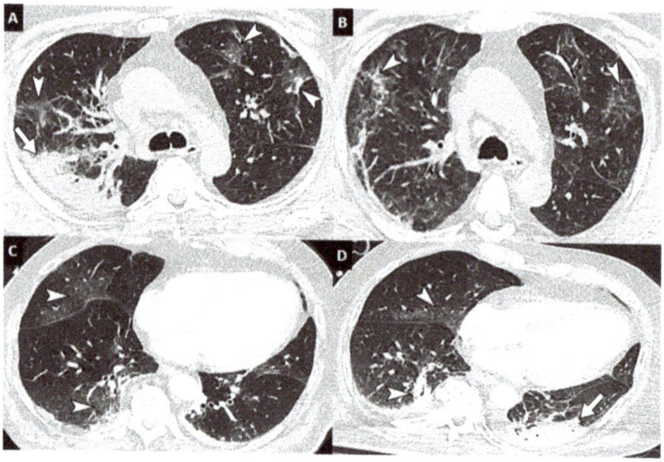

Figure 2. Computed tomography of the chest of patients with COVID-19 with secondary invasive aspergillosis. Unenhanced chest CT in a 59-year-old man with COVID-19 and biological markers of invasive aspergillosis performed at baseline (**A**) and at 12-day follow-up (**B**) showing subpleural ground-glass and reticular opacities presumed to correspond to COVID-19 lesions (arrowheads) as well as a right apical consolidation area presumed to correspond to invasive aspergillosis (arrow). Enhanced chest CT in a 69-year-old man with COVID-19 and biological markers of invasive aspergillosis showing at baseline (**C**) ground-glass opacities (arrowheads), and at 11-day follow-up (**D**) a left postero-basal consolidation presumed to correspond to invasive aspergillosis (arrow). (346-mm field of view, 512 × 512 image matrix, lung window (W1600/L-500 HU)).

Table 7. Outcomes of patients with COVID-19-associated ARDS according to *Aspergillus* status.

Outcomes	All Patients (n = 45)	No Aspergillosis (n = 30)	*Aspergillus* Colonization (n = 8)	Putative/Probable Invasive Aspergillosis (n = 7)	p Value
Duration of mechanical ventilation	17 (9–24)	17 (7–24)	18 (10–21)	18 (12–30)	0.66
Ventilator free days at day 28	11 (4–19)	11 (4–21)	10 (7–18)	10 (0–16)	0.64
Prone positioning ventilation	20 (44)	12 (46)	3 (37.5)	5 (71.4)	0.29
SOFA score on day 7	7 (5–11)	6 (5–10)	8 (7–10)	11 (10–12)	0.01
SOFA score on day 14	7 (2–10)	7 (2–9)	3 (1–7)	9 (2–12)	0.2
ICU length of stay	20 (12–27)	12 (11–23)	23 (16–51)	27 (20–36)	0.02
Death in ICU	6 (13.3)	4 (13.3)	0	2 * (28.6)	0.27

Data are presented as median (IQR: interquartiles), n (%). P values comparing *Aspergillus* colonization, invasive aspergillosis and no aspergillosis groups are tested by Kruskal Wallis (continuous variables) or Chi-square test (categorical variables). Abbreviations: ICU: Intensive Care Unit, SOFA: Sequential Organ Failure Assessment, * 1 putative and 1 probable.

4. Discussion

In France, the global burden of severe fungal infection is estimated at approximately 1,000,000 (1.47%) cases each year [13] and IFD account for a higher risk of mortality in patients with co-morbidities from 9 to 40% [14]. During the COVID-19 pandemic, warning messages considering similarities between Sars-CoV-2 and influenza infections stressed the importance of vigilance towards IFD [15,16]. Local experiences are now published and show high numbers of putative IA [17–22].

The diagnosis of IA still remains challenging because of a wide diversity of underlying conditions and growing number of criteria, particularly biological tools [6]. In deeply immunosuppressed patients, such as neutropenic patients, patients under antineoplastic and prolonged corticosteroid therapy or solid organ transplantation, criteria for classification of IFD and notably IA have recently been revised incorporating *Aspergillus* molecular detection [2]. In ICU, the AspICU algorithm published by Blot et al., [3] is a robust and helpful tool for aspergillosis classification but needs to be more evaluated and even updated. In order to address limitations of the various classification definitions for ICU patients, the ongoing FUNgal infections Definitions in ICU patients (FUNDICU) project aims to develop a standard set of definitions for IFD in critically ill patients [5].

The breaking news of SARS-CoV-2 co-infection urges the need for a critical analysis of the criteria of AspICU algorithm. Indeed, COVID-19 patients, particularly ARDS patients with mechanical ventilation, present with compatible clinical signs as depicted by the algorithm (refractory fever, pleuritic chest pain and rub, dyspnea, hemoptysis and worsening respiratory insufficiency, see [3] for full description) and CT-scan signs are hard to interpret because of COVID-19 CT-scan presentation, leading to absence or very poor discrimination between *Aspergillus* colonization and infection [19,23]. As a result, IA during COVID-19 has been reported with a possible overestimated high prevalence (until 30%), as favorable outcomes have been described in patients who did not receive any antifungal treatment.

In order to have a well-balanced patient management, limiting unnecessary and costly antifungal treatments while not neglecting the life-threatening feature of IA, we included *A. fumigatus* PCR as a monitoring tool for fungal detection in both respiratory and blood samples in addition to classical culture and GM approaches but with some restrictions. As expected, PCR allowed detecting *Aspergillus* in much more respiratory samples. We previously showed that PCR improved the detection of *Aspergillus* in BAL, with a particular added value in ICU patients compared to hematology patients [11]. Furthermore, PCR using in-house but also marketed kits is also capable of identifying specific gene mutations associated with azole resistance [11,24]. Besides, the sensitivity of GM detection in blood is less sensitive in ICU than for patients with hematological malignancies [5]. Here, the higher sensitivity of *Aspergillus* detection also incites us to adopt modified criteria for case definition to gain in specificity. Two major changes were introduced to modify the granularity of the classification: (i) the first one is to combine *Aspergillus* detection in respiratory samples and anti-*Aspergillus* antibody testing, to distinguish chronic colonization (positive serology) from acute massive colonization (negative serology) and (ii) the second is to introduce of obvious biomarkers of angioinvasion (serum GM and blood PCR), similar to those of the EORTC/MSG classification [2]. Of note, the combination of positive culture, positive anti-*Aspergillus* antibody testing and positive GM in the context of chronic respiratory diseases characterized a transition step from chronic pulmonary aspergillosis to probable IA [25,26].

Using this refined classification, we were able to categorize our patients in five classes: no infection, colonization, putative IA, probable IA and proven IA (no case of proven IA in the cohort), with a better relevance than the initial AspICU classification, and better specificity than the AspICU + PCR classification. The decision of antifungal treatment onset was taken according to this modified AspICU classification and the outcome observed gives confidence in this patient management. Of course, the limitation of this work is the relatively small number of patients and should be evaluated on larger cohorts in order to correctly analyze the performance of this alternative. A remaining question is also to determine the place of the serum biomarker (1,3)-β-D-glucan in ICU patients, a question that has recently been raised by Honoré et al. [27]

In conclusion, molecular techniques are now key tools for monitoring IFD, particularly IA as recently updated in the EORTC/MSG definitions, but also *Pneumocystis jirovecii* or mucorales infections. Here, we suggest some adaptations of the AspICU clinical algorithm to gain in sensitivity and specificity. Large multicentric data are needed to confirm this proof of concept study.

Supplementary Materials: The following are available online at http://www.mdpi.com/2309-608X/6/3/105/s1, Table S1: Clinical and biological features of the 9 patients classified as putative aspergillosis according to Blot et al., 2012.

Author Contributions: Conceptualization, J.-P.G., F.R., H.G., J.-M.T. and F.R.-G.; Data curation, J.-P.G., H.G., R.P., M.L. and F.R.-G.; Formal analysis, J.-P.G., F.R., H.G., M.L., J.-M.T. and F.R.-G.; Investigation, J.-P.G., F.R., H.G., K.P., P.L.B., R.P., E.P., S.B., M.L.S., Y.L.T., P.S., M.L. and J.-M.T.; Methodology, J.-P.G., F.R., H.G.and F.R.-G.; Project administration, J.-P.G.; Resources, J.-P.G, F.R., H.G., K.P., P.L.B., R.P., E.P., S.B., M.L.S., Y.L.T., P.S., M.L., J.-M.T. and

F.R.-G.; Software, F.R.; Supervision, J.-P.G. and F.R.-G.; Validation, J.-P.G., Y.L.T. and F.R.-G.; Writing—original draft, J.-P.G. and F.R.-G.; Writing—review & editing, F.R., H.G. and J.-M.T. All authors have read and agreed to the published version of the manuscript.

Funding: This research received no external funding.

Conflicts of Interest: J.-P.G. received funds for communications and congress attendance from Pfizer and Gilead. The other authors declare they have no conflict of interest.

References

1. White, P.L.; Wingard, J.R.; Bretagne, S.; Löffler, J.; Patterson, T.F.; Slavin, M.A.; Barnes, R.A.; Pappas, P.G.; Donnelly, J.P. *Aspergillus* Polymerase Chain Reaction: Systematic Review of Evidence for Clinical Use in Comparison With Antigen Testing. *J. Clin. Microbiol.* **2015**, *61*, 1293–1303. [CrossRef]
2. Donnelly, J.P.; Chen, S.C.; Kauffman, C.A.; Steinbach, W.J.; Baddley, J.W.; Verweij, P.E.; Clancy, C.J.; Wingard, J.R.; Lockhart, S.R.; Groll, A.H.; et al. Revision and Update of the Consensus Definitions of Invasive Fungal Disease From the European Organization for Research and Treatment of Cancer and the Mycoses Study Group Education and Research Consortium. *Clin. Infect. Dis.* **2019**, ciz1008. [CrossRef]
3. Blot, S.; Taccone, F.; Van den Abeele, A.; Meersseman, W.; Brusselaers, W.; Dimopoulos, G.; Paiva, J.; Misset, B.; Rello, J.; Vandewoude, K.; et al. A clinical algorithm to diagnose invasive pulmonary aspergillosis in critically ill patients. *Am. J. Respir. Crit. Care Med.* **2012**, *186*, 56–64. [CrossRef] [PubMed]
4. Bulpa, P.; Bihin, B.; Dimopoulos, G.; Taccone, F.S.; Van den Abeele, A.-M.; Misset, B.; Meersseman, W.; Spapen, H.; Cardoso, T.; Charles, P.-E.; et al. Which algorithm diagnoses invasive pulmonary aspergillosis best in ICU patients with COPD? *Eur. Respir. J.* **2017**, *50*, 1700532. [CrossRef] [PubMed]
5. Bassetti, M.; Giacobbe, D.R.; Grecchi, C.; Rebuffi, C.; Zuccaro, V.; Scudeller, L.; FUNDICU Investigators. Performance of existing definitions and tests for the diagnosis of invasive aspergillosis in critically ill, adult patients: A systematic review with qualitative evidence synthesis. *J. Infect.* **2020**. [CrossRef]
6. Arastehfar, A.; Carvalho, A.; van de Veerdonk, F.L.; Jenks, J.D.; Koehler, P.; Krause, R.; Cornely, O.A.; Perlin, D.S.; Lass-Flörl, C.; Hoenigl, M. COVID-19 Associated Pulmonary Aspergillosis (CAPA)-From Immunology to Treatment. *J. Fungi* **2020**, *6*, 91. [CrossRef]
7. Le Gall, J.R.; Lemeshow, S.; Saulnier, F. A new Simplified Acute Physiology Score (SAPS II) based on a European/North American multicenter study. *JAMA* **1993**, *270*, 2957–2963. [CrossRef]
8. Lambden, S.; Laterre, P.F.; Levy, M.M.; Francois, B. The SOFA score-development, utility and challenges of accurate assessment in clinical trials. *Crit. Care* **2019**, *23*, 374. [CrossRef]
9. Cassagne, C.; Ranque, S.; Normand, A.-C.; Fourquet, P.; Thiebault, S.; Planard, C.; Hendrickx, M.; Piarroux, R. Mould Routine Identification in the Clinical Laboratory by Matrix-Assisted Laser Desorption Ionization Time-Of-Flight Mass Spectrometry. *PLoS ONE* **2011**, *6*. [CrossRef]
10. Normand, A.C.; Becker, P.; Gabriel, F.; Cassagne, C.; Accoceberry, I.; Gari-Toussaint, M.; Hasseine, L.; Geyter, D.D.; Pierard, D.; Surmont, I.; et al. Validation of a New Web Application for Identification of Fungi by Use of Matrix-Assisted Laser Desorption Ionization–Time of Flight Mass Spectrometry. *J. Clin. Microbiol.* **2017**, *55*, 2661–2670. [CrossRef]
11. Guegan, H.; Robert-Gangneux, F.; Camus, C.; Belaz, S.; Marchand, T.; Baldeyrou, M.; Gangneux, J.-P. Improving the diagnosis of invasive aspergillosis by the detection of *Aspergillus* in broncho-alveolar lavage fluid: Comparison of non-culture-based assays. *J. Infect.* **2018**, *76*, 196–205. [CrossRef] [PubMed]
12. Challier, S.; Boyer, S.; Abachin, E.; Berche, P. Development of a Serum-Based Taqman Real-Time PCR Assay for Diagnosis of Invasive Aspergillosis. *J. Clin. Microbiol.* **2004**, *42*, 844–846. [CrossRef] [PubMed]
13. Gangneux, J.-P.; Bougnoux, M.-E.; Hennequin, C.; Godet, C.; Chandenier, J.; Denning, D.W.; Dupont, B. An estimation of burden of serious fungal infections in France. *J. Mycol. Med.* **2016**, *26*, 385–390. [CrossRef] [PubMed]
14. Bitar, D.; Lortholary, O.; Le Strat, Y.; Nicolau, J.; Coignard, B.; Tattevin, P.; Che, D.; Dromer, F. Population-Based Analysis of Invasive Fungal Infections, France, 2001–2010. *Emerg. Infect. Dis.* **2014**, *20*, 1163–1169. [CrossRef] [PubMed]
15. Verweij, P.E.; Gangneux, J.-P.; Bassetti, M.; Brüggemann, R.J.M.; Cornely, O.A.; Koehler, P.; Lass-Flörl, C.; van de Veerdonk, F.L.; Chakrabarti, A.; Hoenigl, M. Diagnosing COVID-19-associated pulmonary aspergillosis. *Lancet Microbe* **2020**, *1*, e53–e55. [CrossRef]

16. Gangneux, J.-P.; Bougnoux, M.-E.; Dannaoui, E.; Cornet, M.; Zahar, J.R. Invasive fungal diseases during COVID-19: We should be prepared. *J. Mycol. Med.* **2020**, *30*, 100971. [CrossRef] [PubMed]
17. Alanio, A.; Dellière, S.; Fodil, S.; Bretagne, S.; Mégarbane, B. Prevalence of putative invasive pulmonary aspergillosis in critically ill patients with COVID-19. *Lancet Respir. Med.* **2020**. [CrossRef]
18. Blaize, M.; Mayaux, J.; Nabet, C.; Lampros, A.; Marcelin, A.-G.; Thellier, M.; Piarroux, R.; Demoule, A.; Fekkar, A. Fatal Invasive Aspergillosis and Coronavirus Disease in an Immunocompetent Patient. *Emerg. Infect. Dis.* **2020**, *26*. [CrossRef]
19. Koehler, P.; Cornely, O.A.; Böttiger, B.W.; Dusse, F.; Eichenauer, D.A.; Fuchs, F.; Hallek, M.; Jung, N.; Klein, F.; Persigehl, T.; et al. COVID-19 associated pulmonary aspergillosis. *Mycoses* **2020**, *63*, 528–534. [CrossRef]
20. Prattes, J.; Valentin, T.; Hoenigl, M.; Talakic, E.; Reisinger, A.C.; Eller, P. Invasive pulmonary aspergillosis complicating COVID-19 in the ICU—A case report. *Med. Mycol. Case Rep.* **2020**. [CrossRef]
21. Van Arkel, A.L.E.; Rijpstra, T.A.; Belderbos, H.N.A.; van Wijngaarden, P.; Verweij, P.E.; Bentvelsen, R.G. COVID-19 Associated Pulmonary Aspergillosis. *Am. J. Respir. Crit. Care Med.* **2020**. [CrossRef] [PubMed]
22. Lescure, F.-X.; Bouadma, L.; Nguyen, D.; Parisey, M.; Wicky, P.-H.; Behillil, S.; Gaymard, A.; Bouscambert-Duchamp, M.; Donati, F.; Hingrat, Q.L.; et al. Clinical and virological data of the first cases of COVID-19 in Europe: A case series. *Lancet Infect. Dis* **2020**, *20*, 697–706. [CrossRef]
23. Rutsaert, L.; Steinfort, N.; Van Hunsel, T.; Bomans, P.; Naesens, R.; Mertes, H.; Dits, H.; Van Regenmortel, N. COVID-19-associated invasive pulmonary aspergillosis. *Ann. Intensive Care* **2020**, *10*, 71. [CrossRef] [PubMed]
24. White, P.L.; Posso, R.B.; Barnes, R.A. Analytical and Clinical Evaluation of the PathoNostics AsperGenius Assay for Detection of Invasive Aspergillosis and Resistance to Azole Antifungal Drugs during Testing of Serum Samples. *J. Clin. Microbiol.* **2015**, *53*, 2115–2121. [CrossRef] [PubMed]
25. Bulpa, P.; Dive, A.; Sibille, Y. Invasive pulmonary aspergillosis in patients with chronic obstructive pulmonary disease. *Eur. Respir. J.* **2007**, *30*, 782–800. [CrossRef]
26. Denning, D.W.; Cadranel, J.; Beigelman-Aubry, C.; Ader, F.; Chakrabarti, A.; Blot, S.; Ullmann, A.J.; Dimopoulos, G.; Lange, C.; on behalf of European Society for Clinical Microbiology and Infectious Diseases and European Respiratory Society. Chronic pulmonary aspergillosis: Rationale and clinical guidelines for diagnosis and management. *Eur. Respir. J.* **2016**, *47*, 45–68. [CrossRef]
27. Honore, P.M.; Barreto Gutierrez, L.; Kugener, L.; Redant, S.; Attou, R.; Gallerani, A.; De Bels, D. Detecting influenza-associated pulmonary aspergillosis by determination of galactomannan in broncho-alveolar lavage fluid and in serum: Should we add (1,3)-beta-D-glucan to improve efficacy. *Crit. Care* **2020**, *24*, 294. [CrossRef]

Journal of *Fungi*

MDPI

Review

COVID-19 Associated Invasive Pulmonary Aspergillosis: Diagnostic and Therapeutic Challenges

Aia Mohamed [1], Thomas R. Rogers [2] and Alida Fe Talento [1,3,*]

[1] Department of Microbiology, Our Lady of Lourdes Hospital Drogheda, A92 VW28 Co. Louth, Ireland; aiamohamed1987@gmail.com
[2] Department of Clinical Microbiology, Trinity College Dublin, St. James's Hospital Campus, D08 NHY1 Dublin, Ireland; rogerstr@tcd.ie
[3] Department of Microbiology, Royal College of Surgeons, Ireland, D02 YN77 Dublin, Ireland
* Correspondence: talenta@tcd.ie; Tel.: +353-419-837-601

Received: 3 July 2020; Accepted: 20 July 2020; Published: 22 July 2020

Abstract: *Aspergillus* co-infection in patients with severe coronavirus disease 2019 (COVID-19) pneumonia, leading to acute respiratory distress syndrome, has recently been reported. To date, 38 cases have been reported, with other cases most likely undiagnosed mainly due to a lack of clinical awareness and diagnostic screening. Importantly, there is currently no agreed case definition of COVID-19 associated invasive pulmonary aspergillosis (CAPA) that could aid in the early detection of this co-infection. Additionally, with the global emergence of triazole resistance, we emphasize the importance of antifungal susceptibility testing in order to ensure appropriate antifungal therapy. Herein is a review of 38 published CAPA cases, which highlights the diagnostic and therapeutic challenges posed by this novel fungal co-infection.

Keywords: COVID-19 pneumonia; invasive pulmonary aspergillosis; diagnosis; multi-triazole resistance; COVID-19 associated invasive pulmonary aspergillosis

1. Introduction

Coronavirus disease 2019 (COVID-19), caused by severe acute respiratory syndrome coronavirus 2 (SARS-CoV-2), is a new viral respiratory infection first reported in Wuhan (Hubei province), China, at the end of 2019 [1]. Since then, more than 10 million confirmed COVID-19 cases, including more than half a million deaths, have been reported [2]. Although infection can vary from asymptomatic to mild upper respiratory infection, it can also lead to a severe pneumonia with acute respiratory distress syndrome (ARDS), requiring critical care and mechanical ventilation [3]. The case fatality rate varies by location and changes over time, and has been reported to be 0.2% in Germany and 7.7% in Italy, with elderly patients noted to have a greater risk of dying [4]. Recently, it was reported that 26% of patients admitted with severe COVID-19 infection died in intensive care [5].

SARS-CoV-2 infection leads to both innate and adaptive immune responses, which include a local immune response, recruiting macrophages and monocytes that respond to the infection, release cytokines, and prime adaptive T and B cell immune responses. In most cases, this process is capable of resolving the infection. However, in some cases, which present as severe COVID-19 infections, a dysfunctional immune response occurs, which can cause significant lung and even systemic pathology [6]. The diffuse alveolar lung damage and dysregulated immune response in severe COVID-19 pneumonia makes these patients vulnerable to secondary infections [6,7]. Viral, bacterial, and fungal co-infections have been reported in COVID-19 patients, and the early diagnosis of these co-infections is important in order to allow for the institution of appropriate antimicrobial therapy [8–10].

COVID-19 associated invasive pulmonary aspergillosis (CAPA) is a recently described syndrome that affects COVID-19 patients with ARDS who require critical care admission. With the global spread of COVID-19, as of 30 June 2020, 38 cases of CAPA have been reported. [11–24]. Here, we review these cases of CAPA so as to highlight the diagnostic and therapeutic challenges posed by this novel fungal co-infection.

2. Coronavirus and Aspergillosis

Coronaviruses are a large group of RNA viruses that infect humans, birds, bats, snakes, mice, and other animals. Seven known human coronaviruses (HCoVs) have been identified with 229E, OC43, NL63, and HKU1 more commonly detected. The first two account for approximately 15–29% of viral respiratory pathogens, with a relatively low virulence in humans [25,26]. The three other strains of HCoVs, namely severe acute respiratory syndrome coronavirus (SARS-CoV), Middle East respiratory syndrome coronavirus (MERS-CoV), and severe acute respiratory syndrome coronavirus 2 (SARS-CoV-2), have a different pathogenic potential, and have been shown to lead to higher mortality rates in humans [26,27].

To date, *Aspergillus* co-infection in patients with coronavirus infections is likely to have been under-diagnosed and under-reported, most likely due to lack of clinical awareness and diagnostic screening [28]. The published literature following severe acute respiratory syndrome (SARS) caused by SARS-CoV-1 has revealed only four cases of invasive aspergillosis (IA), all of which were diagnosed at post-mortem [29–31]. None of the four patients had a previous history of underlying immunocompromise, but they had received corticosteroids, which formed part of the treatment of patients with SARS in 2003. One of these patients was an intensive care physician who received several courses of methylprednisolone. The post-mortem findings in this patient were consistent with disseminated invasive aspergillosis with abscesses in multiple organs [29]. With regards to MERS-CoV, another HCoV that also causes severe respiratory infections, secondary bacterial infections have been reported [32], but a literature search failed to reveal published evidence of *Aspergillus* co-infection. This is most likely explained by the paucity of post-mortems performed on these patients, which were generally not done either for religious and cultural reasons, or to prevent environmental contamination with the subsequent infection of health-care workers [27].

Early reports from China documented *Aspergillus* spp. being isolated from the respiratory samples of patients with COVID-19 pneumonia, however there was no information on its clinical significance, or on the outcome of treatment of these patients [33,34]. Lescure et al. published a case series that detailed the first five imported cases of COVID-19 in France, whereby one of these five patients had severe COVID-19 pneumonia requiring critical care admission, and who was treated with triazoles when *Aspergillus flavus* was isolated from a tracheal aspirate [14].

As of 30 June 2020, 38 cases of CAPA have been reported from several countries, mostly in Europe, but the true incidence of this novel co-infection is unknown. All of the affected patients had been admitted to critical care because of COVID-19 pneumonia and ARDS, requiring ventilatory support. Thirty were males with a mean age of 65.9 (range 38–86, median 70). Table 1 summarizes these 38 cases, their pre-existing co-morbidities, their categorization using published definitions of IA, and their treatment and outcome.

Table 1. Categorization of the 38 published coronavirus disease 2019 (COVID-19) associated invasive pulmonary aspergillosis (CAPA) cases utilizing published definitions for invasive aspergillosis, and their treatment and outcome.

Author/ Country (Prevalence) [Ref]	Age/ Sex	Underlying Conditions	Local/Systemic CS Use	GM (ODI)/Serum BDG (pg/mL)/qPCR	Species (Triazole Susceptibility Pattern)	Expert Panel Case Definition of CAPA [35]	Bulpa et al. [36]	EORTC/MSGERC [37]	*Asp*ICU [38]	Treatment	Outcome
Koehler et al. Single center, retrospective Germany (5/19; 26.3%) [11]	62/F	Cholecystectomy for cholecystitis, arterial hypertension, obesity with sleep apnea, hypercholesterolemia, ex-smoker, COPD (GOLD 2)	Inhaled steroids for COPD	GM Serum negative/GM BALF> 2.5/qPCR BALF = positive	*A. fumigatus* (S) culture from BALF	Probable	Probable	N/A	Putative	VCZ	Died
	70/M	Vertebral disc prolapse left L4/5, ex-smoker	No	GM Serum = 0.7/GM BALF > 2.5/qPCR BALF = positive	Negative culture	Probable	N/A	N/A	N/A	ISA	Died
	54/M	Arterial hypertension, diabetes mellitus, aneurysm coiling	IV CS therapy 0.4 mg/kg/d, total of 13 days)	GM Serum negative/GM BALF > 2.5/qPCR BALF = positive	*A. fumigatus* (S) culture from ETA, ICZ 0.380 μg/mL, VCZ 0.094 μg/mL	Probable	N/A	N/A	Colonisation	CASPO → VCZ	Alive
	73/M	Arterial hypertension, bullous emphysema, smoker, COPD (GOLD 3), previous hepatitis B	Inhaled steroids for COPD	GM Serum negative/qPCR ETA = positive	*A. fumigatus* (S) culture from ETA, ICZ 0.380 μg/mL, VCZ 0.094 μg/mL	N/C	N/C	N/A	Colonisation	VCZ	Died
	54/F	None	No	GM Serum = 1.3 and 2.7qPCR ETA = negative	Negative culture	Probable	N/A	N/A	N/A	CASPO → VCZ	Alive
Alanio et al. Single center prospective France (9/27; 33.3%) [12]	53/M	Hypertension, obesity, ischemic heart disease	Dexamethasone IV 20 mg once daily from day 1 to 5 followed by 10 mg once daily from day 6 to 10	GM Serum = 0.13/GM BALF = 0.89/BDG = 523/qPCR BALF and serum = negative	Negative culture	N/C	N/A	N/A	N/A	None	Alive
	59/F	Hypertension, obesity, diabetes	No	GM Serum = 0.04/GM BALF = 0.03/qPCR BALF = negative	*A. fumigatus*, culture from BALF	Probable	N/A	N/A	Putative	None	Alive
	69/F	Hypertension, obesity	Dexamethasone IV 20 mg once daily from day 1 to 5, followed by 10 mg once daily from day 6 to 10	GM Serum = 0.03/BDG = 7.8/qPCR ETA = 23.9/qPCR serum negative	*A. fumigatus*, culture from ETA	N/C	N/A	N/A	Colonisation	None	Alive

Table 1. *Cont.*

Author/ Country (Prevalence) [Ref]	Age/ Sex	Underlying Conditions	Local/Systemic CS Use	GM (ODI)/Serum BDG (pg/mL)/qPCR	Species (Triazole Susceptibility Pattern)	Expert Panel Case Definition of CAPA [35]	Bulpa et al. [36]	EORTC/MSGERC [37]	*Asp*ICU [38]	Treatment	Outcome
	63/F	Hypertension, diabetes, ischemic heart disease	Dexamethasone IV 20 mg once daily from day 1 to 5, followed by 10 mg once daily from day 6 to 10	GM Serum = 0.51/GM BALF= 0.15/BDG = 105/qPCR BALF and serum = negative	Negative culture	Probable	N/A	N/A	N/A	None	Died
	43/M	Asthma with steroid use history	No	GM Serum = 0.04/GM BALF = 0.12/BDG = 7/qPCR BALF and serum = negative	*A. fumigatus*, culture from BALF	Probable	N/A	N/A	Putative	None	Alive
	79/M	Hypertension	Dexamethasone IV 20 mg once daily from day 1 to 5, followed by 10 mg once daily from day 6 to 10	GM Serum = 0.02/GM BALF = 0.05/BDG = 23/qPCR BALF = 34.5/qPCR serum = negative	*A. fumigatus*, culture from BALF	Probable	N/A	N/A	Putative	None	Alive
	77/M	Hypertension, asthma	Dexamethasone iv 20 mg once daily from day 1 to 5, followed by 10 mg once daily from day 6 to 10	GM Serum = 0.37/GM BALF = 3.91/BDG = 135/qPCR BALF = 29/qPCR serum = negative	*A. fumigatus*, culture from BALF	Probable	N/A	N/A	Putative	VCZ	Died
	75/F	Hypertension, diabetes	Dexamethasone iv 20 mg once daily from day 1 to day 5, followed by 10 mg once daily from day 6 to day 10	GM Serum = 0.37 GM BALF = 0.36 BDG = 450 qPCR BALF = 31.7 qPCR serum = Negative	*A. fumigatus*, culture from BALF	Probable	N/A	N/A	Putative	CASPO	Died
	47/M	Multiple myeloma with steroid therapy	No	GM Serum = 0.09 BDG = 14 qPCR ETA and serum = Negative	*A. fumigatus*, culture from ETA	N/C	N/A	Probable	Colonisation	None	Died

Table 1. *Cont.*

Author/ Country (Prevalence) [Ref]	Age/ Sex	Underlying Conditions	Local/Systemic CS Use	GM (ODI)/Serum BDG (pg/mL)/qPCR	Species (Triazole Susceptibility Pattern)	Expert Panel Case Definition of CAPA [35]	Bulpa et al. [36]	EORTC/MSGERC [37]	*Asp*ICU [38]	Treatment	Outcome
Van Arkel et al. Single center prospective Netherlands (6/31; 19.4%) [17]	83/M	Cardiomyopathy	Prednisolon 0.13 mg/kg/day for 28 days pre-admission	GM Serum = 0.4	*A. fumigatus*, culture from ETA	N/C	N/A	N/A	Colonisation	VCZ + ANID (5/6) L-AmB (1/6)	Died
	67/M	COPD (GOLD 3), Post RTx NSCLC 2014	Prednisolon 0.37 mg/kg/day for 2 days pre-admission	Not reported	*A. fumigatus*, culture from ETA	N/C	Possible	N/A	Colonisation		Died
	75/M	COPD (GOLD 2a)	No	GM BALF = 4.0	*A. fumigatus*, culture from BALF	Probable	Probable	N/A	Putative		Died
	43/M	None	No	GM Serum = 0.1 GM BALF = 3.8	Negative culture	Probable	N/A	N/A	N/A		Alive
	57/M	Bronchial asthma	Fluticason 1.94 mcg/kg/day for 1 month pre-admission	GM Serum = 0.1 GM BALF = 1.6	*A. fumigatus*. culture from BALF	Probable	N/A	N/A	Putative		Died
	58/M	None	No	Not reported	*Aspergillus spp.* culture from sputum	N/C	N/A	N/A	Colonisation		Alive
Rutsaert et al. Single center prospective Belgium (7/20; 35%) [13]	86/M	Hypercholesterinemia	No	GM serum = 0.1	*A. flavus* culture from ETA	N/C	N/A	N/A	Colonisation	None	Died
	38/M	Obesity, hypercholesterinemia	No	GM serum = 0.3 GM BALF > 2.8	*A. fumigatus* culture from BALF	Proven	N/A	Proven	Proven	VCZ, ISA	Alive
	62/M	Diabetes	No	GM serum = 0.2 GM BALF = 2	*A. fumigatus* culture from BALF	Proven	N/A	Proven	Proven	VCZ	Died
	73/M	Diabetes, obesity, hypertension, hypercholesterinemia	No	GM serum = 0.1 GM BALF > 2.8	*A. fumigatus* culture from BALF	Proven	N/A	Proven	Proven	VCZ	Alive
	77/M	Diabetes, chronic kidney disease, hypertension, pemphigus foliaceus	No	GM serum = 0.1 GM BALF = 2.79	*A. fumigatus* culture from BALF	Proven	N/A	Proven	Proven	VCZ	Alive
	55/M	HIV, hypertension, hypercholesterinemia	No	GM serum = 0.80 GM BALF = 0.69	Negative culture	Probable	N/A	N/A	N/A	VCZ, ISA	Died
	75/M	Acute myeloid leukemia	No	GM BALF = 2.63	*A. fumigatus* culture from BALF	Probable	N/A	N/A	Putative	VCZ	Died

Table 1. *Cont.*

Author/ Country (Prevalence) [Ref]	Age/ Sex	Underlying Conditions	Local/Systemic CS Use	GM (ODI)/Serum BDG (pg/mL)/qPCR	Species (Triazole Susceptibility Pattern)	Expert Panel Case Definition of CAPA [35]	Bulpa et al. [36]	EORTC/MSGERC [37]	*Asp*ICU [38]	Treatment	Outcome
Blaize et al. Case Report France (1) [19]	74/M	Myelodysplastic syndrome, $CD8^+$ T-cell lymphocytosis, Hashimoto's thyroiditis, hypertension, benign prostatic hypertrophy	No	Serum GM, BDG and qPCR negative, GM First ETA = negative First qPCR ETA = positive Second qPCR ETA = positiveDirect smear of the second ETA = branched septate hyphae	*A. fumigatus*, culture of second ETA	N/C	N/A	N/A	Colonisation	None	Died
Lescure et al. Case Series France (1/5; 20%) [14]	80/M	Thyroid cancer 2010 (patient presented with ARDS)	No	Not reported	*A. flavus*, culture from ETA	N/C	N/A	N/A	Colonisation	VCZ → ISA	Died
Antinori et al. Case Report Italy (1) [18]	73/M	Diabetes, hypertension, obesity, hyperthyroidism, atrial fibrillation	No	GM Serum = 8.6 qPCR from paraffin block tissue = positive	*A. fumigatus*, culture from BALF	Proven	N/A	Proven	Proven	L-AmB → ISA	Died
Prattes et al. Case Report Austria (1) [20]	70/M	COPD (GOLD 2), obstructive sleep apnea syndrome, insulin-dependent type 2 diabetes with end organ damage, arterial hypertension, coronary heart disease, obesity	Inhaled Budesonide (400 mg per day)	GM Serum = negative BDG = negative LFD positive from ETA	*A. fumigatus*, (S) culture from ETA VCZ = 0.125 µg/mL	N/C	N/A	N/A	Colonisation	VCZ	Died
Lahmer et al. Case Series Germany (2) [22]	80/M	Suspected pulmonary fibrosis	No	GM Serum = 1.5 GM BALF = 6.3	*A. fumigatus*, culture from BALF	Probable	N/A	N/A	Putative	L-AmB	Died
	70/M	None	No	GM Serum = negative GM BALF = 6.1	*A. fumigatus*, culture from BALF	Probable	N/A	N/A	Putative	L-AmB	Died
Meijer et al. Case Report Netherlands (1) [21]	74/F	Polyarthrosis, reflux, stopped smoking 20 years ago	No	GM serum = persistently < 0.5 GM ETA ≥ 3 BDG = 1590	*A. fumigatus*, culture from ETA $(R)^{TR34/L98H}$ICZ = 16 µg/mL, VCZ = 2 µg/mL, and POSA = 0.5 µg/mL	N/C	N/A	N/A	Colonisation	VCZ + CASPO → Oral VCZ → L-AmB	Died
Mohamed et al. Case Report Ireland (1) [23]	66/M	Obesity, diabetes mellitus, hypertension, stopped smoking >10 years ago	No	GM serum = 1.1 GM ETA = 5.5 BDG = 202 qPCR ETA–*A. fumigati* complex	*A. fumigatus* culture from ETA (R) $^{TR34/L98H}$ICZ ≥ 32 µg/mL, VCZ = 2 µg/mL and POSA = 1 µg/mL	Probable	N/A	N/A	Colonisation	L-AmB	Died

Table 1. *Cont.*

Author/ Country (Prevalence) [Ref]	Age/ Sex	Underlying Conditions	Local/Systemic CS Use	GM (ODI)/Serum BDG (pg/mL)/qPCR	Species (Triazole Susceptibility Pattern)	Expert Panel Case Definition of CAPA [35]	Bulpa et al. [36]	EORTC/MSGERC [37]	*Asp*ICU [38]	Treatment	Outcome
Sharma et al. Case Report Australia (1) [24]	66/F	Hypertension, recent ex-smoker of 20 pack years	No	Not done	*A. fumigatus* from ETA	N/C	N/A	N/A	Colonisation	VCZ	Alive
Santana et al. Case Report Brazil (1) [15]	71/M	Hypertension, diabetes mellitus, chronic kidney disease	No	GM stored blood 4.29 qPCR of lung tissue, Sequencing identified *Aspergillus penicillioides*	Not done	Proven	N/A	Proven	Proven	None	Died
Ferreira et al. Case Report France (1) [16]	56/M	Hypertension, diabetes mellitus, hyperlipidemia, obesity	Fluticasone propionate/ salmeterol inhaler, Dexamethasone IV 20 mg × 7 days	GM serum First sample = 0.07, Second sample = 0.05 BDG First sample = 10.4, Second sample ≤ 7.8 qPCR ETA 26.3 qPCR serum negative	*A. fumigatus*, culture from ETA $(R)^{TR34/L98H}$ICZ = >8 µg/mL, VCZ = 2 µg/mL, ISA 4 ug/mL and POSA = 0.5 µg/mL	N/C	N/A	N/A	Colonisation	None	Died

Legend: N/A, not applicable; N/C, not classifiable; M, male; F, female; IV intravenous; CS corticosteroids; BALF bronchoalveolar lavage fluid; ETA, endotracheal aspirate; GM, galactomannan; ODI, optical density index; qPCR, quantitative polymerase chain reaction; BDG, 1-3 β-d-glucan; LFD, *Aspergillus* lateral flow device; ICZ itraconazole; VCZ, voriconazole; ISA, isavuconazole; POSA, posaconazole; CASPO, caspofungin; L-AmB, liposomal amphotericin-B; S, susceptible; r, resistant; COPD, chronic obstructive pulmonary disease; GOLD, Global Initiative for Chronic Obstructive Lung Disease; RTx, radiotherapy; NSCLC, non-small cell lung cancer; ARDS, adult respiratory distress syndrome.

3. Diagnosis of CAPA

The diagnosis of proven IA requires culture or histopathologic findings from biopsy or sterile site samples [37,38]. There are only six proven cases from the 38 reviewed here. One patient was suspected to have CAPA pre-mortem, when *A. fumigatus* was isolated from bronchoalveolar lavage fluid (BALF) and the serum galactomannan (GM) optical density index (ODI) was 8.6. Despite antifungal therapy (AFT), the patient succumbed to the infection, and the diagnosis of CAPA was confirmed at post-mortem. Another patient was diagnosed at post-mortem with histopathologic findings of fungal hyphae and spores in the lung tissue, further confirmed by nucleotide sequencing and identified as *A. penicillioides*. A stored peripheral blood sample revealed a GM ODI of 4.290 [15]. The other four proven cases were diagnosed by histopathological examination of the biopsy material taken from a bronchoscopy of the suspicious tracheobronchial lesions [13]. However, most patients with severe COVID-19 pneumonia are usually critically ill and hemodynamically unstable, which will preclude performing invasive procedures, such as bronchoscopy with a lavage or a lung biopsy. Furthermore, bronchoscopy is not recommended in patients with COVID-19 because of the risks this aerosol generating procedure imposes on both the patient and the attending healthcare worker, unless deemed life-saving [39]. According to current guidelines that are specific to different patient populations, the diagnosis of probable or putative invasive aspergillosis (IA) is made using a composite of host factors, clinical features, and mycological evidence of aspergillus infection [36–38]. Most patients with CAPA, including those with proven IA, did not have the host factors described for IA by the European Organization for Research and Treatment of Cancer and the Mycoses Study Group Education and Research Consortium (EORTC/MSGERC). Severe viral pneumonia is not considered a risk factor for invasive pulmonary aspergillosis, even though the structural damage as well as the dysregulated immune response can predispose to secondary co-infection with *Aspergillus* sp. [6,7]. An alternative diagnostic approach is to apply the clinical algorithm, which has been validated for the diagnosis of IA in patients in critical care [38], with severe COVID-19 infection, and the isolation of *Aspergillus* sp. from a BALF as the entry criteria. Recently, a panel of experts proposed case definitions for influenza-associated pulmonary aspergillosis that might also be considered for the classification of CAPA patients, while awaiting further histopathological studies that will provide more insight into the interaction between *Aspergillus* and SARS-CoV-2-infected lungs [35]. Patients with confirmed severe COVID-19 infection and pulmonary infiltrates on chest imaging should trigger investigation for the presence of *Aspergillus* infection by the culture of respiratory samples and/or the detection of GM either in serum or BALF, if and when bronchoscopy is performed. However, serum GM has a low sensitivity in non-neutropenic patients [40], and bronchoscopy may not be feasible. Endotracheal aspirates (ETA) are a potentially safer alternative investigative option, as their collection does not involve an aerosol generating procedure; however, their use for GM detection has not been validated. In previous reports, culturing *Aspergillus* spp. from ETA samples has been interpreted as colonization only, however when considered in conjunction with the clinical presentation and biomarkers, such as serum GM, this may suggest IA [41,42]. Of the 38 reported CAPA cases reviewed here, 16 and 14 patients had an *Aspergillus* sp. isolated from BALF and ETA samples, respectively, and another patient had *Aspergillus* sp. cultured from a sputum sample, with *A. fumigatus* being the most common species identified. The BALF/ETA GM indices were ≥1 in 16 of 23 patients, and the serum GM ODI was ≥0.5 in only 9 of 33 cases. New point-of-care tests for the detection of the *Aspergillus*-specific antigen or for GM from serum or BALF may also be useful as early evidence of CAPA in critically ill COVID-19 patients [43–47]. One patient with CAPA was reported to have the *Aspergillus* specific antigen detected from an ETA utilizing a lateral flow device [20]. The diagnostic performance of this lateral flow assay in the early diagnosis of IA in patients with severe influenza and/or COVID-19 is currently being investigated (ISRCTN51287266) [48]. Serum 1-3 β-D-glucan (BDG), a panfungal marker, was positive in 6 of 14 CAPA cases where BDG was reported. Although non-specific for *Aspergillus* infection, this biomarker is included as an indirect mycological criterion in the EORTC/MSGERC definitions; therefore, a positive BDG may help to support the diagnosis of CAPA [37] with an improved diagnostic performance when there are ≥2 positive results [49]. The detection of *Aspergillus* DNA using real-time PCR is another modality that may support the diagnosis of probable IA [37]. *Aspergillus* DNA was detected in 13 of 19 CAPA patients where real-time quantitative PCR was performed on either respiratory or serum samples.

The typical "halo sign" associated with IPA in neutropenic patients is uncommonly seen in non-neutropenic patients with IPA, where radiological imaging may show varying patterns from multiple pulmonary nodules to various non-specific findings, which include consolidation, cavitation, pleural effusions, ground glass opacities, tree-in-bud opacities, and atelectasis [37,50]. High resolution computed tomography (CT) is preferred to other imaging, such as chest radiographs [37,50]. Of the 38 reported CAPA cases, CT was performed in 15, where one patient was noted to have a reverse halo sign [20], six patients had ground glass opacities and varying sizes and numbers of nodules noted [11], while the others had findings "typical" of COVID-19 pneumonia. Patients with severe COVID-19 pneumonia in critical care are often clinically unfit for additional imaging, adding to the difficulty in interpreting the significance of the isolation of an *Aspergillus* sp. from upper respiratory tract samples.

Excluding the six proven CAPA cases, 18 of the remaining 32 cases reviewed here fulfilled the case definition of probable CAPA, as suggested by the expert panel [35]; 11 had putative IPA utilizing the *Asp*ICU criteria [38]; and one had probable CAPA utilizing EORTC/MSGERC definitions [37]. Two patients with chronic obstructive pulmonary disease (COPD) could be classified as probable CAPA, following definitions by Bulpa et al. for COPD patients [36]. We emphasize that definitions published by the EORTC/MSGERC are recommended only for research purposes, and should not be used for clinical decision making [37]. Perhaps a more pragmatic approach to the diagnosis of CAPA would be, in the setting of a patient with severe COVID-19 pneumonia in critical care, to combine ≥2 mycological criteria to include the following:

1. GM detection from serum/BALF/ETA
2. Isolation of *Aspergillus* sp. from BALF/ETA/sputa
3. Serum BDG detection
4. Detection of *Aspergillus* DNA by real time PCR in blood or respiratory samples

This approach may aid in the early institution of antifungal therapy.

4. Antifungal Treatment Strategies for CAPA

The clinical suspicion, or proven diagnosis, of *Aspergillus* co-infection should trigger the initiation of empiric or targeted antifungal therapy, respectively, even though its efficacy is not established. We note that only 13 of the 38 reported cases survived their infection, and those dying succumbed to multi-organ failure and sepsis. International treatment guidelines recommend the triazoles voriconazole or isavuconazole as the first-line treatment of IA [50,51]. The emergence of multi-triazole resistance in *A. fumigatus* challenges the efficacy of triazoles in the successful treatment of IPA [52–54], particularly in areas of high prevalence, and their use in such cases is associated with increased mortality [55]. Triazole resistance in *A. fumigatus* is causally linked to the use of triazole compounds that are structurally similar to those used in medical practice, as agricultural fungicides, or less commonly to prolonged triazole use in individual patients [54]. The former mechanism of resistance typically affects azole näive patients, and is characterized by elevated minimum inhibitory concentrations (MIC) of itraconazole, voriconazole, posaconazole, and isavuconazole. This underlines the importance of antifungal susceptibility testing (AFST) either through phenotypic or genotypic methods to detect triazole resistance, which will help direct the choice of treatment. Although cultures are generally known to have a poor diagnostic sensitivity [56], the ability to culture *Aspergillus* sp. will allow for the determination of MICs for triazoles. Recently, a four-well triazole resistance screening plate was validated for *A. fumigatus*, which can be useful in laboratories that do not have the capacity to perform the recommended broth microdilution methods for AFST [57–59]. Genotypic testing that utilizes molecular assays has also been evaluated to detect *Aspergillus* spp. and the common mutations associated with triazole resistance directly from clinical samples [60–63], which will allow for the rapid detection of a marker of resistance and guide treatment options. Twenty-two of the 38 CAPA cases reviewed here received a triazole-based AFT regimen either alone or in combination with an echinocandin or liposomal amphotericin B. Only seven cases reported susceptibility results based on either phenotypic testing and/or the detection of common mutations associated with triazole resistance using molecular techniques. Three cases were reported to be caused by a triazole-resistant *A. fumigatus*, all of which were confirmed to have the *cyp51A* TR_{34} L98H mutation [16,21,23]. Knowledge of the local epidemiology of triazole resistance is important to help guide the choice of therapy while awaiting susceptibility results. It has been recommended that for areas with triazole resistance rates of >10%, voriconazole-echinocandin combination therapy or liposomal amphotericin B should be used as the initial therapy [52]. However, in many countries, there are no surveillance systems in place to determine the prevalence of triazole resistance in *A. fumigatus*, which is known to be the most common *Aspergillus* spp. causing IA, as has also been observed in the CAPA cases reported to date.

Rutsaert et al. from the Netherlands reported administering prophylactic aerosolised liposomal amphotericin-B to all COVID-19 patients on mechanical ventilation in critical care, after they identified a cluster of seven CAPA cases, four of which were proven. Antifungal prophylaxis formed part of a multi-faceted management of this cluster, which also included the bi-weekly GM screening of serum and BALF, if and when a bronchoscopy was performed. High-efficiency particulate air filters were also installed in their critical care unit. The authors reported that no further cases were detected after the implementation of these measures at the time of writing. The rationale for prospective trials would need to be determined in order to establish whether antifungal prophylaxis in severe COVID-19 cases is indicated. A clinical trial of posaconazole prophylaxis for the prevention of pulmonary aspergillosis in patients with severe influenza (NCT03378479) is currently ongoing and this will provide data on the effectiveness of this approach, at least for influenza [64].

New antifungal agents with novel modes of action are in the pipeline so as to address the problem of antifungal resistance, which threatens the effectiveness of the few agents currently being used to treat invasive fungal disease [65]. Clinical trials are ongoing for three new antifungal agents, namely, ibrexafungerp (NCT03672292) [66], olorofim (NCT03583164) [67], and fosmanogepix (NCT04240886) [68]. Ibrexafungerp, which is structurally similar to echinocandins, inhibits fungal β-1,3-glucan synthase with activity against triazole-resistant *Aspergillus* sp. Olorofim and fosmanogepix have different novel targets, which are fungal dihydroorotate dehydrogenase, an important enzyme in fungal DNA synthesis, and the inhibition of fungal enzyme Gwt1 inactivating modification of mannoproteins, which is an important component in maintaining fungal cell wall integrity, respectively [69,70]. All three agents have activity against *Aspergillus* spp., including *A. fumigatus*, which may impact positively on the future management of patients with IA and more specifically CAPA.

5. Conclusions

This review has highlighted the diagnostic and therapeutic challenges of CAPA, a newly identified fungal co-infection in patients with severe COVID-19. We underline the pitfalls of the current definitions of IA applied to these patients, and the need for further evaluation of the usefulness of the culture and detection of fungal antigens from upper respiratory tract specimens in the diagnosis of IA. Additionally, given the global emergence of triazole resistance in *Aspergillus* spp., performing AFST by phenotypic methods and/or the detection of mutations associated with antifungal resistance by genotypic methods is crucial to allow for the timely institution of appropriate antifungal therapy, and will provide valuable information on the prevalence of triazole resistance in *A. fumigatus* and other *Aspergillus* spp. for surveillance purposes. Furthermore, properly designed trials are needed in order to determine the optimum therapeutic approach for patients with CAPA.

Author Contributions: A.M., T.R.R. and A.F.T. contributed equally in the literature review, writing and editing of the manuscript. All authors have read and agreed to the published version of the manuscript.

Funding: There was no external funding for this work.

Conflicts of Interest: A.M. has no conflict of interests. T.R. Rogers received grants and personal fees from Gilead Sciences, personal fees and educational meeting support from Pfizer Healthcare Ireland, and personal fees from Menarini Pharma outside the submitted work. A.F. Talento received grant and personal fees from Gilead Sciences, and personal fees from Pfizer Healthcare Ireland outside the submitted work.

References

1. Zhu, N.; Zhang, D.; Wang, W.; Li, X.; Yang, B.; Song, J.; Zhao, X.; Huang, B.; Shi, W.; Lu, R.; et al. A novel coronavirus from patients with pneumonia in China, 2019. *N. Engl. J. Med.* **2020**, *382*, 727–733. [CrossRef]
2. Coronavirus Disease 2019 (COVID-19) Situational Report. Available online: https://www.who.int/docs/default-source/coronaviruse/situation-reports/20200702-covid-19-sitrep-164.pdf?sfvrsn=ac074f58_2 (accessed on 2 July 2020).
3. Cevik, M.; Bamford, C.; Ho, A. COVID-19 pandemic—A focused review for clinicians. *Clin. Microbiol. Infect.* **2020**. [CrossRef]
4. Mortality Risk of COVID-19. Available online: https://ourworldindata.org/mortality-risk-covid (accessed on 2 July 2020).
5. Grasselli, G.; Zangrillo, A.; Zanella, A.; Antonelli, M.; Cabrini, L.; Castelli, A.; Cereda, D.; Coluccello, A.; Foti, G.; Fumagalli, R.; et al. Baseline Characteristics and Outcomes of 1591 Patients Infected With SARS-CoV-2 Admitted to ICUs of the Lombardy Region, Italy. *JAMA* **2020**, 1–8. Available online: http://www.ncbi.nlm.nih.gov/pubmed/32250385 (accessed on 2 July 2020).
6. Tay, M.Z.; Poh, C.M.; Rénia, L.; MacAry, P.A. Ng LFP The trinity of COVID-19: Immunity, inflammation and intervention. *Nat. Rev. Immunol.* **2020**, *20*, 363–374. [CrossRef]
7. Chuan, Q.; Luoqi, Z.; Ziwei, H.; Shuoqi, Z.; Sheng, Y.; Yu, T.; Cuihong, X.; Ke, M.; Ke, S.; Wei, W.; et al. Dysregulated immune response in patients with COVID-19 in Wuhan China. *Clin. Infect. Dis.* **2020**. [CrossRef]
8. Lansbury, L.; Lim, B.; Baskaran, V.; Lim, W.S. Co-infections in people with COVID-19: A systematic review and meta-analysis. *J. Infect.* **2020**. [CrossRef] [PubMed]
9. Rawson, T.M.; Moore, L.S.P.; Zhu, N.; Ranganathan, N.; Skolimowska, K.; Gilchrist, M.; Satta, G.; Cooke, G.; Holmes, A. Bacterial and fungal co-infection in individuals with coronavirus: A rapid review to support COVID-19 antimicrobial prescribing. *Clin. Infect. Dis.* **2020**. [CrossRef] [PubMed]
10. Lai, C.-C.; Wang, C.-Y.; Hsueh, P.-R. Co-infections among patients with COVID-19: The need for combination therapy with non-anti-SARS-CoV-2 agents? *J. Microbiol. Immunol. Infect.* **2020**. [CrossRef]
11. Koehler, P.; Cornely, O.A.; Böttiger, B.W.; Dusse, F.; Eichenauer, D.A.; Fuchs, F.; Hallek, M.; Jung, N.; Klein, F.; Persigehl, T.; et al. COVID-19 associated pulmonary aspergillosis. *Mycoses* **2020**, *63*, 528–534. [CrossRef]
12. Alanio, A.; Dellière, S.; Fodil, S.; Bretagne, S. High prevalence of putative invasive pulmonary aspergillosis in critically ill COVID-19 patients. *Lancet Respir. Med.* **2020**, *8*, e48–e49. [CrossRef]
13. Rutsaert, L.; Steinfort, N.; Van Hunsel, T.; Bomans, P.; Naesens, R.; Mertes, H.; Dits, H.; Van Regenmortel, N. COVID-19-associated invasive pulmonary aspergillosis. *Ann. Intensiv. Care* **2020**, *10*, 71. Available online: http://www.ncbi.nlm.nih.gov/pubmed/32488446 (accessed on 2 July 2020). [CrossRef]
14. Antinori, S.; Rech, R.; Galimberti, L.; Castelli, A.; Angeli, E.; Fossali, T.; Bernasconi, D.; Covizzi, A.; Bonazzetti, C.; Torre, A.; et al. Clinical and virological data of the first cases of COVID-19 in Europe: A case series. *Lancet Infect. Dis.* **2020**, *20*, 697–706. [CrossRef]
15. Santana, M.F.; Pivoto, G.; Alexandre, M.A.A.; Baja-da-Silva, D.C.; da Silva Barba, M.; Val, F.A.; Brito-Sousa, J.D.; Melo, G.C.; Monteiro, W.M.; Souza, J.V.B.; et al. Confirmed Invasive Pulmonary Aspergillosis and COVID-19: The value of postmortem findings to support antemortem management. *J. Brazilian Soc. Trop. Med.* **2020**, *53*, e20200401. [CrossRef] [PubMed]
16. Ferreira, T.G.; Saade, A.; Alanio, A.; Bretagne, S.; Castro, R.A.; De Hamane, S.; Azoulay, E.; Bredin, S. Recovery of a triazole-resistant Aspergillus fumigatus in respiratory specimen of COVID-19 patient in ICU—A case report. *Med. Mycol. Case Rep.* **2020**. Available online: https://doi.org/10.1016/j.mmcr.2020.06.006 (accessed on 2 July 2020).
17. Van Arkel, A.L.E.; Rijpstra, T.A.; Belderbos, H.N.A.; van Wijngaarden, P.; Verweij, P.E.; Bentvelsen, R.G. COVID-19 Associated Pulmonary Aspergillosis. *Am. J. Respir. Crit. Care Med.* **2020**, 1–10. [CrossRef] [PubMed]

18. Antinori, S.; Rech, R.; Galimberti, L.; Castelli, A.; Angeli, E.; Fossali, T.; Bernasconi, D.; Covizzi, A.; Bonazzetti, C.; Torre, A.; et al. Invasive pulmonary aspergillosis complicating SARS-CoV-2 pneumonia: A diagnostic challenge. *Travel Med. Infect. Dis.* **2020**, 101752. [CrossRef] [PubMed]
19. Blaize, M.; Mayaux, J.; Nabet, C.; Lampros, A.; Marcelin, A.-G.; Thellier, M.; Piarroux, R.; Demoule, A.; Fekkar, A. Fatal Invasive Aspergillosis and Coronavirus Disease in an Immunocompetent Patient. *Emerg. Infect. Dis.* **2020**, *26*, 1636–1637. [CrossRef] [PubMed]
20. Prattes, J.; Valentin, T.; Hoenigl, M.; Talakic, E.; Reisinger, A.C.; Eller, P. Invasive pulmonary aspergillosis complicating COVID-19 in the ICU—A case report. *Med. Mycol. Case Rep.* **2020**. [CrossRef] [PubMed]
21. Meijer, E.F.J.; Dofferhoff, A.S.M.; Hoiting, O.; Buil, J.B.; Meis, J.F. Azole-Resistant COVID-19-Associated Pulmonary Aspergillosis in an Immunocompetent Host: A Case Report. *J. Fungi* **2020**, *6*, 79. [CrossRef]
22. Lahmer, T.; Rasch, S.; Spinner, C.; Geisler, F.; Schmid, R.M.; Huber, W. Invasive pulmonary aspergillosis in severe severe coronavirus disease 2019 pneumonia. *Clin. Microbiol. Infect.* **2020**. [CrossRef]
23. Mohamed, A.; Hassan, T.; Trzos-Grzybowska, M.; Thomas, J.; Quinn, A.; O'Sullivan, M.; Griffin, A.; Rogers, T.R.; Talento, A.F. Multi-triazole-resistant Aspergillus fumigatus and SARS-CoV-2 co-infection: A lethal combination. *Med. Mycol. Case Rep.* **2020**. [CrossRef]
24. Sharma, A.; Hofmeyr, A.; Bansal, A.; Thakkar, D.; Lam, L.; Harrington, Z.; Bhonagiri, D. COVID-19 associated pulmonary aspergillosis (CAPA): An Australian case report. *Med. Mycol. Case Rep.* **2020**. [CrossRef]
25. Li, G.; Fan, Y.; Lai, Y.; Han, T.; Li, Z.; Zhou, P.; Pan, P.; Wang, W.; Hu, D.; Liu, X.; et al. Coronavirus infections and immune responses. *J. Med. Virol.* **2020**, *92*, 424–432. [CrossRef] [PubMed]
26. Yang, Y.; Peng, F.; Wang, R.; Guan, K.; Jiang, T.; Xu, G.; Sun, J.; Chang, C. The deadly coronaviruses: The 2003 SARS pandemic and the 2020 novel coronavirus epidemic in China. *J. Autoimmun.* **2020**, *109*, 102434. [CrossRef] [PubMed]
27. Memish, Z.A.; Perlman, S.; Van Kerkhove, M.D.; Zumla, A. Middle East respiratory syndrome. *Lancet* **2020**, *395*, 1063–1077. [CrossRef]
28. Thompson, I.G.R.; A Cornely, O.; Pappas, P.G.; Patterson, T.F.; Hoenigl, M.; Jenks, J.D.; Clancy, C.J.; Nguyen, M.H. On behalf of the MSG (MSG) and EC of MM (ECMM). Invasive aspergillosis as an underrecognized superinfection in COVID-19. *Open Forum Infect. Dis.* **2020**. [CrossRef]
29. Wang, H.; Ding, Y.; Li, X.; Yang, L.; Zhang, W.; Kang, W. Fatal Aspergillosis in a Patient with SARS Who Was Treated with Corticosteroids. *N. Engl. J. Med.* **2003**, *349*, 507–508. [CrossRef]
30. Wang, H.-J.; Ding, Y.-Q.; Xu, J.; Li, X.; Li, X.-F.; Yang, L.; Zhang, W.; Geng, J.; Shen, H.; Cai, J.-J.; et al. Death of a SARS case from secondary aspergillus infection. *Chin. Med. J.* **2004**, *117*.
31. Hwang, D.M.; Chamberlain, D.W.; Poutanen, S.M.; E Low, D.; Asa, S.L.; Butany, J. Pulmonary pathology of severe acute respiratory syndrome in Toronto. *Mod. Pathol.* **2004**, *18*, 1–10. [CrossRef]
32. Arabi, Y.M.; Deeb, A.M.; Al-hameed, F.; Mandourah, Y.; Mady, A.; Alraddadi, B.; Almotairi, A.; Al, K.; Abdulmomen, A.; Qushmaq, I.; et al. Macrolides in critically ill patients with Middle East Respiratory Syndrome. *Int. J. Infect. Dis.* **2019**, *81*, 184–190. [CrossRef]
33. Chen, N.; Zhou, M.; Dong, X.; Qu, J.; Gong, F.; Han, Y.; Qiu, Y.; Wang, J.; Liu, Y.; Wei, Y.; et al. Epidemiological and clinical characteristics of 99 cases of 2019 novel coronavirus pneumonia in Wuhan, China: A descriptive study. *Lancet* **2020**, *395*, 507–513. [CrossRef]
34. Yang, X.; Yu, Y.; Xu, J.; Shu, H.; Xia, J.; Liu, H.; Wu, Y.; Zhang, L.; Yu, Z.; Fang, M.; et al. Clinical course and outcomes of critically ill patients with SARS-CoV-2 pneumonia in Wuhan, China: A single-centered, retrospective, observational study. *Lancet Respir. Med.* **2020**, *2600*, 1–7. [CrossRef]
35. Verweij, P.; Rijnders, B.J.A.; Brüggemann, R.J.M.; Azoulay, E.; Bassetti, M.; Blot, S.; Calandra, T.; Clancy, C.J.; Cornely, O.A.; Chiller, T.; et al. Review of influenza-associated pulmonary aspergillosis in ICU patients and proposal for a case definition: An expert opinion. *Intensiv. Care Med.* **2020**, 1–12. (In Press) [CrossRef]
36. Bulpa, P.; Dive, A.; Sibille, Y. Invasive pulmonary aspergillosis in patients with chronic obstructive pulmonary disease. *Eur. Respir. J.* **2007**, *30*, 782–800. [CrossRef] [PubMed]
37. Donnelly, J.P.; Chen, S.C.; Kauffman, C.A.; Steinbach, W.J.; Baddley, J.W.; Verweij, P.E.; Clancy, C.J.; Wingard, J.R.; Lockhart, S.R.; Groll, A.H.; et al. Revision and Update of the Consensus Definitions of Invasive Fungal Disease From the European Organization for Research and Treatment of Cancer and the Mycoses Study Group Education and Research Consortium. *Clin. Infect. Dis.* **2019**. [CrossRef] [PubMed]

38. Blot, S.I.; Taccone, F.S.; Van Den Abeele, A.M.; Bulpa, P.; Meersseman, W.; Brusselaers, N.; Dimopoulos, G.; Paiva, J.A.; Misset, B.; Rello, J.; et al. A Clinical Algorithm to Diagnose Invasive Pulmonary Aspergillosis in Critically Ill Patients. *Am. J. Respir. Crit. Care Med.* **2012**, *186*, 56–64. Available online: http://www.embase.com/search/results?subaction=viewrecord&from=export&id=L36516539 (accessed on 2 July 2020). [CrossRef] [PubMed]
39. Wahidi, M.M.; Shojaee, S.; Lamb, C.R.; Ost, D.; Maldonado, F.; Eapen, G.; Caroff, D.A.; Stevens, M.P.; Ouellette, D.R.; Lilly, C.; et al. The Use of Bronchoscopy During the COVID-19 Pandemic. *Chest* **2020**, 1–14. [CrossRef] [PubMed]
40. Meersseman, W.; Lagrou, K.; Maertens, J.; Wilmer, A.; Hermans, G.; Vanderschueren, S.; Spriet, I.; Verbeken, E.; Van Wijngaerden, E. Galactomannan in bronchoalveolar lavage fluid, a tool for diagnosing aspergillosis in intensive care unit patients. *Am. J. Respir. Crit. Care Med.* **2008**, *177*, 27–34. [CrossRef]
41. Vandewoude, K.H.; Blot, S.I.; Depuydt, P.; Benoit, D.; Temmerman, W.; Colardyn, F.; Vogelaers, D. Clinical relevance of Aspergillus isolation from respiratory tract samples in critically ill patients. *Crit. Care* **2006**, *10*, R31. [CrossRef]
42. Koulenti, D.; Vogelaers, D.; Blot, S. What's new in invasive pulmonary aspergillosis in the critically ill. *Intensiv. Care Med.* **2014**, *40*, 723–726. [CrossRef]
43. Lass-Flörl, C.; Lo Cascio, G.; Nucci, M.; dos Santos, M.C.; Colombo, A.L.; Vossen, M.; Willinger, B. Respiratory specimens and the diagnostic accuracy of Aspergillus lateral flow assays (LFA-IMMY^{TM}): Real-life data from a multicentre study. *Clin. Microbiol. Infect.* **2019**, *25*, 1563.e1–1563.e3.
44. Eigl, S.; Prattes, J.; Lackner, M.; Willinger, B.; Spiess, B.; Reinwald, M.; Selitsch, B.; Meilinger, M.; Neumeister, P.; Reischies, F.; et al. Multicenter evaluation of a lateral-flow device test for diagnosing invasive pulmonary aspergillosis in ICU patients. *Crit. Care* **2015**, *19*, 1–10. [CrossRef]
45. Willinger, B.; Lackner, M.; Lass-Florl, C.; Prattes, J.; Posch, V.; Selitsch, B.; Eschertzhuber, S.; Honigl, K.; Koidl, C.; Sereinigg, M.; et al. Bronchoalveolar lavage lateral-flow device test for invasive pulmonary aspergillosis in solid organ transplant patients: A semiprospective multicenter study. *Transplantation* **2014**, *98*, 898–902. [CrossRef] [PubMed]
46. Hsu, J.L.; Ruoss, S.J.; Bower, N.D.; Lin, M.; Holodniy, M.; Stevens, D.A. Diagnosing invasive fungal disease in critically ill patients. *Crit. Rev. Microbiol.* **2011**, *37*, 277–312. Available online: http://www.embase.com/search/results?subaction=viewrecord&from=export&id=L362711815 (accessed on 2 July 2020). [CrossRef] [PubMed]
47. White, P.L.; Price, J.S.; Posso, R.; Cutlan-Vaughan, M.; Vale, L.; Backx, M. Evaluation of the Performance of the IMMY sona Aspergillus Galactomannan Lateral Flow Assay When Testing Serum To Aid in Diagnosis of Invasive Aspergillosis. *J. Clin. Microbiol.* **2020**, *58*, e00053-20. [CrossRef] [PubMed]
48. Youngs, J.; Bicanic, T. *Aspergillosis in Patients with Severe Influenza or Coronavirus*. ISRCTN51287266. Available online: http://www.isrctn.com/ISRCTN51287266 (accessed on 2 July 2020). [CrossRef]
49. Talento, A.F.; Dunne, K.; Joyce, E.A.; Palmer, M.; Johnson, E.; White, P.L.; Springer, J.; Loeffler, J.; Ryan, T.; Collins, D.; et al. A prospective study of fungal biomarkers to improve management of invasive fungal diseases in a mixed specialty critical care unit. *J. Crit. Care* **2017**, *40*. [CrossRef]
50. Ullmann, A.J.; Aguado, J.M.; Arikan-Akdagli, S.; Denning, D.W.; Groll, A.H.; Lagrou, K.; Lass-Flörl, C.; Lewis, R.E.; Munoz, P.; Verweij, P.E.; et al. Diagnosis and management of Aspergillus diseases: Executive summary of the 2017 ESCMID-ECMM-ERS guideline. *Clin. Microbiol. Infect.* **2018**, *24* (Suppl. 1), e1–e38. Available online: http://linkinghub.elsevier.com/retrieve/pii/S1198743$\times$1830051X. (accessed on 16 May 2018).
51. Patterson, T.F.; Thompson, G.R.; Denning, D.W.; Fishman, J.A.; Hadley, S.; Herbrecht, R.; Kontoyiannis, D.P.; Marr, K.A.; Morrison, V.A.; Nguyen, M.H.; et al. Practice guidelines for the diagnosis and management of aspergillosis: 2016 update by the infectious diseases society of America. *Clin. Infect. Dis.* **2016**, *63*, e1–e60. [CrossRef]
52. Verweij, P.E.; Ananda-Rajah, M.; Andes, D.; Arendrup, M.C.; Bruggemann, R.J.; Chowdhary, A.; Cornely, O.A.; Denning, D.W.; Groll, A.H.; Izumikawa, K.; et al. International expert opinion on the management of infection caused by azole-resistant Aspergillus fumigatus. *Drug Resist. Updat.* **2015**, *21–22*, 30–40. [CrossRef]
53. Sharpe, A.R.; Lagrou, K.; Meis, J.F.; Chowdhary, A.; Lockhart, S.R.; Verweij, P.E. Triazole resistance surveillance in Aspergillus fumigatus. *Med. Mycol.* **2018**, *56*, S83–S92. [CrossRef]
54. Verweij, P.E.; Mellado, E.; Melchers, W.J. Multiple-Triazole–Resistant Aspergillosis. *N. Engl. J. Med.* **2007**, *356*, 1481–1483. [CrossRef]

55. Resendiz-Sharpe, A.; Mercier, T.; Lestrade, P.P.A.; Van Der Beek, M.T.; Von Dem Borne, P.A.; Cornelissen, J.J.; De Kort, E.; Rijnders, B.J.A.; Schauwvlieghe, A.F.A.D.; Verweij, P.E.; et al. Prevalence of voriconazole-resistant invasive aspergillosis and its impact on mortality in haematology patients. *J. Antimicrob. Chemother.* **2019**, *74*, 2759–2766. [CrossRef]
56. Schelenz, S.; Barnes, R.A.; Barton, R.C.; Cleverley, J.R.; Lucas, S.B.; Kibbler, C.C.; Denning, D.W. British Society for Medical Mycology best practice recommendations for the diagnosis of serious fungal diseases. *Lancet Infect. Dis.* **2015**, *15*, 461–474. [CrossRef]
57. Van der Linden, J.W.M.; Arendrup, M.C.; Van der Lee, H.A.L.; Melchers, W.J.G.; Verweij, P.E. Azole containing agar plates as a screening tool for azole resistance of Aspergillus fumigatus. *Mycoses* **2009**, *52*, 19.
58. Arendrup, M.C.; E Verweij, P.; Mouton, J.W.; Lagrou, K.; Meletiadis, J. Multicentre validation of 4-well azole agar plates as a screening method for detection of clinically relevant azole-resistant Aspergillus fumigatus. *J. Antimicrob. Chemother.* **2017**, *72*, 3325–3333. [CrossRef] [PubMed]
59. Tsitsopoulou, A.; Posso, R.; Vale, L.; Bebb, S.; Johnson, E.; White, P.L. Determination of the Prevalence of Triazole Resistance in Environmental Aspergillus fumigatus Strains Isolated in South Wales, UK. *Front. Microbiol.* **2018**, *9*, 1–8. [CrossRef]
60. Zhao, Y.; Garnaud, C.; Brenier-Pinchart, M.P.; Thiébaut-Bertrand, A.; Saint-Raymond, C.; Camara, B.; Hamidfar, R.; Cognet, O.; Maubon, D.; Cornet, M.; et al. Direct molecular diagnosis of aspergillosis and CYP51A profiling from respiratory samples of french patients. *Front. Microbiol.* **2016**, *7*, 1–7. [CrossRef] [PubMed]
61. Denning, D.W.; Park, S.; Lass-Florl, C.; Fraczek, M.G.; Kirwan, M.; Gore, R.; Smith, J.; Bueid, A.; Moore, C.B.; Bowyer, P.; et al. High-frequency triazole resistance found in nonculturable aspergillus fumigatus from lungs of patients with chronic fungal disease. *Clin. Infect. Dis.* **2011**, *52*, 1123–1129. [CrossRef] [PubMed]
62. Torelli, R.; Sanguinetti, M.; Moody, A.; Pagano, L.; Caira, M.; De Carolis, E.; Fuso, L.; De Pascale, G.; Bello, G.; Antonelli, M.; et al. Diagnosis of invasive aspergillosis by a commercial real-time PCR assay for Aspergillus DNA in bronchoalveolar lavage fluid samples from high-risk patients compared to a galactomannan enzyme immunoassay. *J. Clin. Microbiol.* **2011**, *49*, 4273–4278. Available online: http://www.embase.com/search/results?subaction=viewrecord&from=export&id=L363013871 (accessed on 25 June 2020).
63. White, P.L.; Posso, R.B.; Barnes, R.A. Analytical and Clinical Evaluation of the PathoNostics AsperGenius Assay for Detection of Invasive Aspergillosis and Resistance to Azole Antifungal Drugs during Testing of Serum Samples. *J. Clin. Microbiol.* **2015**, *53*, 2115–2121. [CrossRef]
64. Posaconazole for the Prevention of Influenza-associated Aspergillosis in Critically Ill Patients (POSA-FLU) NCT03378479. Available online: https://clinicaltrials.gov/ct2/show/NCT03378479. (accessed on 28 June 2020).
65. Rauseo, A.M.; Coler-Reilly, A.; Larson, L.; Spec, A. Hope on the horizon: Novel fungal treatments in development. *Open Forum Infect. Dis.* **2020**, *7*, 1–19. [CrossRef] [PubMed]
66. Study to Evaluate the Safety and Efficacy of the Coadministration of Ibrexafungerp (SCY-078) With Voriconazole in Patients With Invasive Pulmonary Aspergillosis (SCYNERGIA). Available online: https://clinicaltrials.gov/ct2/show/NCT03672292. (accessed on 28 June 2020).
67. Evaluate F901318 Treatment of Invasive Fungal Infections in Patients Lacking Treatment Options (FORMULA-OLS). Available online: https://clinicaltrials.gov/ct2/show/NCT03583164. (accessed on 28 June 2020).
68. An Open-label Study of APX001 for Treatment of Patients With Invasive Mold Infections Caused by Aspergillus Species or Rare Molds AEGIS. Available online: https://clinicaltrials.gov/ct2/show/NCT04240886 (accessed on 28 June 2020).
69. Van Daele, R.; Spriet, I.; Wauters, J.; Maertens, J.; Mercier, T.; Van Hecke, S.; Brüggemann, R. Antifungal drugs: What brings the future? *Med. Mycol.* **2019**, *57*, S328–S343. [CrossRef]
70. Gintjee, T.J.; Donnelley, M.A.; Thompson, G.R. Aspiring Antifungals: Review of Current Antifungal Pipeline Developments. *J. Fungi.* **2020**, *6*, 28. [CrossRef]

Journal of *Fungi*

MDPI

Case Report

Azole-Resistant COVID-19-Associated Pulmonary Aspergillosis in an Immunocompetent Host: A Case Report

Eelco F. J. Meijer [1,2,3], Anton S. M. Dofferhoff [3,4], Oscar Hoiting [5], Jochem B. Buil [1,2] and Jacques F. Meis [1,2,3,6,*]

1 Department of Medical Microbiology, Radboud University Medical Center, 6500HB Nijmegen, The Netherlands; Eelco.Meijer@radboudumc.nl (E.F.J.M.); Jochem.Buil@radboudumc.nl (J.B.B.)
2 Center of Expertise in Mycology Radboudumc/CWZ, 6532 SZ Nijmegen, The Netherlands
3 Department of Medical Microbiology and Infectious Diseases, Canisius Wilhelmina Hospital (CWZ), 6532 SZ Nijmegen, The Netherlands; A.Dofferhoff@cwz.nl
4 Department of Internal Medicine, Canisius Wilhelmina Hospital (CWZ), 6532 SZ Nijmegen, The Netherlands
5 Department of Intensive Care Medicine, Canisius Wilhelmina Hospital (CWZ), 6532 SZ Nijmegen, The Netherlands; O.Hoiting@cwz.nl
6 Bioprocess Engineering and Biotechnology Graduate Program, Federal University of Paraná, Curitiba 81531-970, PR, Brazil
* Correspondence: jacques.meis@gmail.com; Tel.: +31-24-365-7514

Received: 26 May 2020; Accepted: 4 June 2020; Published: 6 June 2020

Abstract: COVID-19-associated pulmonary aspergillosis (CAPA) is a recently described disease entity affecting patients with severe pulmonary abnormalities treated in intensive care units. Delays in diagnosis contribute to a delayed start of antifungal therapy. In addition, the emergence of resistance to triazole antifungal agents puts emphasis on early surveillance for azole-resistant *Aspergillus* species. We present a patient with putative CAPA due to *Aspergillus fumigatus* with identification of a triazole-resistant isolate during therapy. We underline the challenges faced in the management of these cases, the importance of early diagnosis and need for surveillance given the emergence of triazole resistance.

Keywords: SARS-CoV-2; co-infection; pulmonary aspergillosis; ICU; azole-resistant *Aspergillus*; *Aspergillus fumigatus*; CAPA; TR_{34}L98H

1. Introduction

There have been suggestions that coronavirus disease 2019 (COVID-19) might increase the risk of superinfections [1] and, particularly, invasive pulmonary aspergillosis (IPA) co-infection [2]. COVID-19-associated pulmonary aspergillosis (CAPA) is a recently described disease entity affecting patients in intensive care unit (ICUs) with severe pulmonary abnormalities. Small cohorts of 31 patients in the Netherlands [3], 27 patients in France [4] and 19 patients in Germany [5] have been published, showing CAPA rates of 19.4%, 33% and 26%, respectively. An additional two fatal cases of CAPA were recently reported [6,7]. The numbers resemble what has been observed in influenza, where influenza in ICU patients has been identified as an independent risk factor for invasive pulmonary aspergillosis and which is associated with an even higher mortality rate than IPA alone [8]. In addition, in the Netherlands, an estimated 11.3% of cases with invasive aspergillosis are infected with an azole-resistant isolate [9], potentially increasing mortality to 50–100% [10]. We present the first case of azole-resistant *Aspergillus fumigatus* in a SARS-CoV-2-positive immunocompetent patient admitted to the ICU.

2. Case Report and Results

A 74-year-old patient was admitted because of respiratory insufficiency amid the COVID-19 crisis. Eleven days prior to admission, she had been suffering from fever (38.5 °C) and a dry cough. Three days after symptom onset, she developed diarrhea. Her medical history included complaints of reflux and pain due to arthrosis of the hip and knees, for which she uses a proton-pump inhibitor and a nonsteroidal anti-inflammatory drug pantoprazol and etoricoxib, respectively. She stopped smoking 20 years ago and was healthy and fit otherwise. Patient characteristics can be found in Table 1. This study, "Clinical course and prognostic factors for COVID-19" with project identification code CWZ-nr 027-2020, was approved in March 20202 by the Canisius Wilhelmina Hospital medical ethics committee and patient informed consent was acquired antemortem with opt out possibility.

Table 1. Patient characteristics

Gender		Female
Age (years)		74
Medical history		Reflux, polyarthrosis, stopped smoking 20 years ago
Medication		Pantoprazol (PPI) and Etoricoxib (NSAID)
Underlying immuno-compromising condition		None
Initial symptoms		Fever, dry cough, dyspneic, diarrhea
ARDS	Prone positioning	Yes
	vvECMO	No
Acute renal failure		Yes, continuous venovenous hemofiltration (CVVH)
IPA definition	EORTC/MSG criteria	N/A
	(modified) AspICU algorithm	N/A

At presentation to the emergency department, she had been feeling progressively dyspneic for two days. On physical examination, her oxygenation was 82%, with 28 breaths per minute in room air, pulmonary wheezing and an extended expiration. Oxygenation improved to 94% with 5 L O_2 via a nasal cannula, but she desaturated during speech. Her BMI was 27.7 (80 kg) and her temperature 37.8 °C. No other aberrant observations on physical examination were made. Her Glasgow Coma Scale was 15 and her ECG was normal. Her C-reactive protein (CRP) was 214 mg/L, and other laboratory findings included slightly elevated leucocytes (12.6×10^9 /L) and neutrophils (8.4×10^9 /L), elevated liver enzymes (alkaline phosphatase 528 U/L; GGT 376 U/L; AST 76 U/L; LD 745 U/L), slightly elevated pro-calcitonin (0.25 μg/L; <0.5 μg/L not suggestive of bacterial infection), increased ferritin (1442 μg/L), and normal electrolyte, glucose and renal function. SARS-CoV-2 nasopharyngeal and throat swabs were taken. A low-dose chest CT demonstrated extensive centralized and peripheral bilateral ground glass opacities with left-sided consolidations and bilateral fibrotic bands without pleural effusions and vascular enlargement (Figure 1). The CO-RADS score was 5 and CT-severity score was 24 out of 25 [11].

Because of the high probability of SARS-CoV-2 infection, chloroquine treatment was started (600 mg and 300 mg on day 1, 300 mg q12h days 2–5), which was national policy at the time. The SARS-CoV-2 PCR of a nasopharyngeal swab was positive (Ct 30.59; E gene [12]). Blood cultures remained negative, as were nasopharynx bacterial cultures taken at admission. The patient was subsequently admitted to our general inpatient respiratory ward. An overview of her hospital course is depicted in Figure 2.

The CRP remained highly stable over the following days at around 200 mg/L with a range of 192–214. However, the patient needed increasing oxygenation with a non-rebreathing mask. Empirical treatment of a suspected bacterial superinfection was started with ceftriaxone i.v. 2000 mg q24h. Five days after admission, the maximum (15 L O_2) oxygenation with the non-rebreathing mask became insufficient and the patient was admitted to the ICU for respiratory support and intensive monitoring.

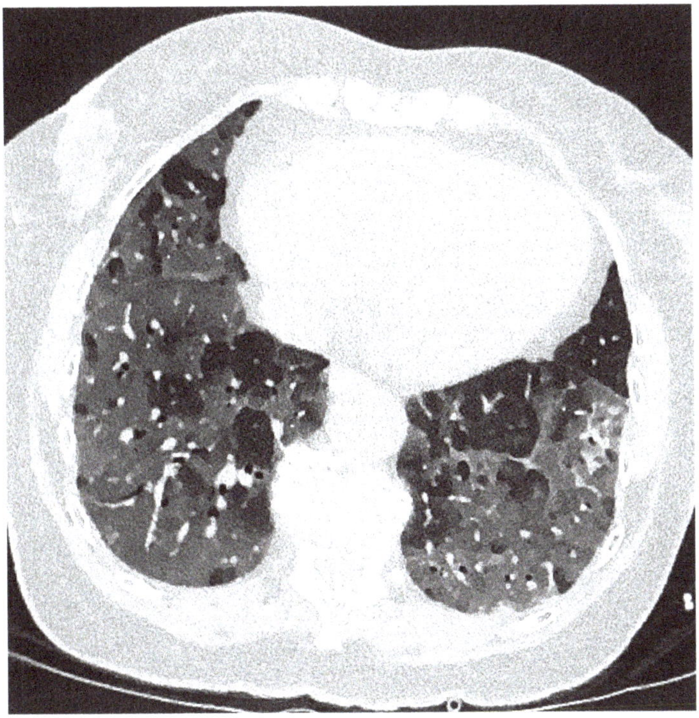

Figure 1. Low-dose chest CT showing extensive centralized and peripheral bilateral ground glass opacities with left-sided consolidations and bilateral fibrotic bands. No pleural effusion. No vascular enlargement and no specific suggestions of aspergillosis.

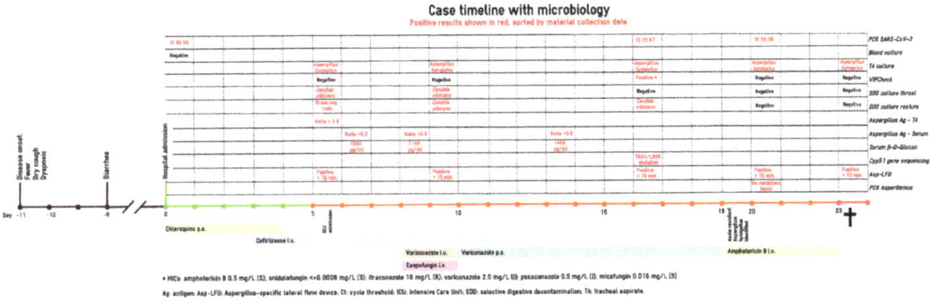

Figure 2. Case timeline with microbiology.

In the ICU, HFNO (high-flow nasal oxygen therapy) and selective digestive decontamination (SDD) were initiated, which includes ceftriaxone i.v. 2000 mg q24h for 4 days and a combined oral non-absorbable suspension of amphotericin B, colistin and tobramycin q6h. In this patient, ceftriaxone was continued de facto for another 4 days. Routine bacterial and fungal (peri-anal, throat and tracheal aspirate) surveillance cultures were done twice weekly in adherence with our local SDD policy [13]. Within a few hours after admission to the ICU, her blood oxygenation became insufficient with HFNO at FiO2 100% and 60 L/min flow. Therefore, she was sedated, intubated and put on a mechanical ventilator. A CT angiography of the chest was performed which demonstrated significant bilateral pulmonary emboli. Anticoagulants (enoxaparine anti-factor Xa) were initiated in therapeutic dosages. Pressure control ventilation was required with the patient in prone position. Because of the need for increasing noradrenaline dosages during circulatory shock, hydrocortisone 100 mg q8h was initiated and continued for five days. Cardiac ultrasound showed a minor tricuspid insufficiency but no major pathology.

Aspergillus fumigatus was recovered from high-volume tracheal aspirate cultures [14] obtained at ICU admission. Aspergillus galactomannan (Platelia Aspergillus; Bio-Rad, Marnes-La-Coquette, France) ratio at this time was >3.0 (positive) in a tracheal aspirate and β-D-glucan (Fungitell assay; Associates of Cape Cod Inc., East Falmouth, MA, USA) in serum was 1590 pg/mL (positive), after which a putative diagnosis of CAPA was made. Serum galactomannan remained negative (<0.5) in three subsequent samples. Voriconazole i.v. 6 mg/kg q12h was started in addition to caspofungin i.v. 70 mg q24h until the VIPcheck (Mediaproducts BV, Groningen, The Netherlands), used to detect azole resistance, was negative. MICs determined with broth microdilution using CLSI methodology of the *A. fumigatus* isolate were as follows: amphotericin B 0.5 mg/L, micafungin and anidulafungin <0.016 mg/L, itraconazole 1 mg/L, voriconazole 0.25 mg/L, and posaconazole 0.063 mg/L. Voriconazole was switched to oral administration of 200 mg q12h with discontinuation of caspofungin. During SDD, bacterial cultures remained negative throughout her stay in the ICU.

On day 6 after admission (day 2 at the ICU), continuous venovenous hemofiltration was initiated because of rapidly progressive acute renal failure. *A. fumigatus* was persistently cultured from tracheal aspirate samples during voriconazole treatment and β-D-glucan levels remained positive with 1149 and 1458 pg/μl, at 1 and 6 days (day 8 and 13 after hospital admission) of voriconazole therapy, respectively. Voriconazole serum therapeutic drug monitoring was performed as recommended [15], with therapeutic concentrations of 4.72 mg/L, 2.78 mg/L and 1.43 mg/L at day 13, 15 and 17, respectively.

The respiratory situation improved marginally in the subsequent 7 days but declined steadily thereafter. Pressure support and pressure control ventilation were alternated between days 12 and 19 and attempts to return the patient to a supine position failed several times. After 7 days, *A. fumigatus* grew on the itraconazole and voriconazole wells of the second VIPcheck on day 19 (tracheal aspirate culture). MICs of this *A. fumigatus* isolate were as follows: amphotericin B 0.5 mg/L, anidulafungin and micafungin <0.016 mg/L, itraconazole 16 mg/L, voriconazole 2 mg/L and posaconazole 0.5 mg/L. Voriconazole treatment was changed to liposomal amphotericin B 200 mg q24h. Subsequent *cyp51A* gene sequencing identified a TR_{34}/L98H mutation, probably responsible for the observed azole resistance. On day 22, ventilation and oxygenation of the patient deteriorated further without further treatment options and therapy was discontinued on day 23. An autopsy was not performed.

3. Discussion

We report the first case of azole-resistant CAPA, which occurred in an immunocompetent host during ICU support without a previous history of azole therapy. The *A. fumigatus cyp51A* gene TR_{34}/L98H mutation found in this patient has been well described as an environmentally acquired mutation [16], which is in line with data from clinical studies where two-thirds of patients with azole-resistant infections had no history of azole pretreatment [10]. This case underscores the importance of early diagnosis and the need for resistance surveillance, comparable to what has been described in influenza patients [9,17], given the emergence of triazole resistance [18,19].

The sensitivity for detection of resistance in primary cultures with the VIPcheck plate depends on the number of *A. fumigatus* colonies that are tested, as clinical cultures may contain both mixed azole-susceptible and azole-resistant isolates during an infection [20]. We suspect that *A. fumigatus* isolated in the first tracheal aspirate was already a mixed culture but was missed in initial fungal cultures due to abundance of azole-susceptible *A. fumigatus* spores. Molecular detection could have given a suggestion to the presence of a mixed culture [21] but PCR could not be performed due to absence of material. The TR_{34}/L98H had a phenotype with high itraconazole MIC (>16 mg/L) and low voriconazole MIC (2 mg/L), similar to strains which have been described only recently in the Netherlands [22].

IPA is known to be problematic to diagnose in the non-neutropenic ICU host [23]. Regardless of the compelling evidence for CAPA in this patient, the EORTC/MSGERC [24] host criteria for invasive fungal disease were not met, nor did the patient meet the AspICU algorithm because we tested tracheal aspirates instead of bronchoalveolar lavage (BAL) fluid [25]. This is in line with findings from other groups, where CAPA patients did not meet the EORTC/MSGERC host criteria either [3–6]. In addition, the American Association for Bronchology and Interventional Pulmonology (AABIP) has issued a statement advising against routine bronchoscopy in COVID-19 patients, as it poses substantial risk to patients and staff [26]. BAL should only be considered in intubated patients if upper respiratory samples are negative and BAL would significantly change clinical management. Tracheal aspirate cultures, as performed twice weekly in our patient, repeatedly identified *A. fumigatus* as the only micro-organism present. In the first positive culture, five colonies were tested for resistance with the VIPcheck plate as is recommended to exclude azole resistance [15]. When surveillance cultures of tracheal aspirates were persistently cultured positive with *A. fumigatus* during voriconazole therapy, we suspected the selection of resistant isolates which were probably already present in the first samples, albeit in undetectable numbers. An autopsy to confirm IPA was not done.

Serum galactomannan testing has been shown to be a fairly sensitive diagnostic tool (70%) in neutropenic patients with pathology-proven invasive aspergillosis [27,28]. However, in patients who are non-neutropenic, serum galactomannan sensitivity of around 25% has been reported [27], which may explain the low number of serum galactomannan positive findings in recently published case reports [6,7] and case series [3–5]. The role of β-D-glucan and the *Aspergillus*-specific lateral flow device (LFD) as an adjunct to the diagnosis of IPA in COVID-19 is not yet clear [2,23]. Serum β-D-glucan was persistently strongly positive in this patient over the course of a week. The specificity for invasive fungal disease of β-D-glucan testing in a mixed ICU population has been shown to be high (86%), with two consecutive positive results [29] compared to those with only fungal colonization and no invasive fungal disease. In addition, multiple other studies report a good sensitivity for the diagnosis of invasive aspergillosis in critically ill patients [30–34]. BAL β-D-glucan in the ICU setting is, however, not recommended, due to its poor specificity and confounders causing false positive results [35].

The LFD is particularly interesting in the ICU due to its short turnaround time. It has demonstrated a higher sensitivity but lower specificity in BAL fluids compared to galactomannan [36] and β-D-glucan [37] in IPA-probable and proven immunocompromised patients. In the ICU setting, however, LFD is suggested to have a lower sensitivity but comparable specificity to galactomannan testing in BAL fluids [35,38]. Noteworthily, a negative predictive value of >96% has been reported in the ICU setting [39]. We used the OLM lateral flow device (AspLFD) on sequential patient tracheal aspirates, yielding positive results on all samples confirming the positive galactomannan result. Although suitable for its negative predictive value or as an additional diagnostic measure, further evaluation of lateral flow technology in critically ill patients is warranted.

Altogether, we describe the clinical course of the first reported patient with azole-resistant CAPA. The contribution of *A. fumigatus* to this fatal COVID-19 course is highly likely, although autopsy was not performed, as in all previously reported CAPA cases [3–7].

Author Contributions: Conceptualization, J.F.M. and A.S.M.D.; formal analysis, E.F.J.M.; investigation, O.H. and J.B.B.; resources, J.F.M.; data curation, A.S.M.D. and O.H.; writing—original draft preparation, E.M. and J.F.M.; writing—review and editing, A.S.M.D., O.H., J.B.B.; supervision, J.F.M. All authors have read and agreed to the published version of the manuscript.

Funding: This research received no external funding.

Acknowledgments: We thank Paul E Verweij M.D. for helpful discussions.

Conflicts of Interest: The authors declare no conflict of interest.

References

1. Clancy, C.J.; Nguyen, M.H. COVID-19, superinfections and antimicrobial development: What can we expect? *Clin. Infect. Dis.* **2020**. [CrossRef] [PubMed]
2. Verweij, P.E.; Gangneux, J.-P.; Bassetti, M.; Brüggemann, R.J.M.; Cornely, O.A.; Koehler, P.; Lass-Flörl, C.; van de Veerdonk, F.L.; Chakrabarti, A.; Hoenigl, M. Diagnosing COVID-19-associated pulmonary aspergillosis. *Lancet Microbe* **2020**. [CrossRef]
3. van Arkel, A.L.E.; Rijpstra, T.A.; Belderbos, H.N.A.; van Wijngaarden, P.; Verweij, P.E.; Bentvelsen, R.G. COVID-19 associated pulmonary aspergillosis. *Am. J. Respir. Crit. Care Med.* **2020**. [CrossRef] [PubMed]
4. Alanio, A.; Dellière, S.; Fodil, S.; Bretagne, S.; Mégarbane, B. High prevalence of putative invasive pulmonary aspergillosis in critically Ill COVID-19 patients. *Lancet Respir. Med.* **2020**. [CrossRef]
5. Koehler, P.; Cornely, O.A.; Bottiger, B.W.; Dusse, F.; Eichenauer, D.A.; Fuchs, F.; Hallek, M.; Jung, N.; Klein, F.; Persigehl, T.; et al. COVID-19 associated pulmonary aspergillosis. *Mycoses* **2020**, *63*, 528–534. [CrossRef]
6. Marion, B.; Julien, M.; Cécile, N.; Alexandre, L.; Anne-Geneviève, M.; Marc, T.; Renaud, P.; Alexandre, D.; Arnaud, F. Fatal invasive aspergillosis and coronavirus disease in an immunocompetent patient. *Emerg. Infect. Dis.* **2020**, *26*. [CrossRef]
7. Prattes, J.; Valentin, T.; Hoenigl, M.; Talakic, E.; Reisinger, A.C.; Eller, P. Invasive pulmonary aspergillosis complicating COVID-19 in the ICU - A case report. *Med. Mycol. Case Rep.* **2020**. [CrossRef]
8. Schauwvlieghe, A.; Rijnders, B.J.A.; Philips, N.; Verwijs, R.; Vanderbeke, L.; Van Tienen, C.; Lagrou, K.; Verweij, P.E.; Van de Veerdonk, F.L.; Gommers, D.; et al. Invasive aspergillosis in patients admitted to the intensive care unit with severe influenza: A retrospective cohort study. *Lancet Respir. Med.* **2018**, *6*, 782–792. [CrossRef]
9. Buil, J.B.; Meijer, E.F.J.; Denning, D.W.; Verweij, P.E.; Meis, J.F. Burden of serious fungal infections in the Netherlands. *Mycoses* **2020**, *63*, 625–631. [CrossRef]
10. Meis, J.F.; Chowdhary, A.; Rhodes, J.L.; Fisher, M.C.; Verweij, P.E. Clinical implications of globally emerging azole resistance in *Aspergillus fumigatus*. *Philos. Trans. R Soc. Lond. B Biol. Sci.* **2016**, *371*. [CrossRef]
11. Prokop, M.; van Everdingen, W.; van Rees Vellinga, T.; Quarles van Ufford, J.; Stoger, L.; Beenen, L.; Geurts, B.; Gietema, H.; Krdzalic, J.; Schaefer-Prokop, C.; et al. CO-RADS - A categorical CT assessment scheme for patients with suspected COVID-19: Definition and evaluation. *Radiology* **2020**, 201473. [CrossRef] [PubMed]
12. Corman, V.M.; Landt, O.; Kaiser, M.; Molenkamp, R.; Meijer, A.; Chu, D.K.; Bleicker, T.; Brunink, S.; Schneider, J.; Schmidt, M.L.; et al. Detection of 2019 novel coronavirus (2019-nCoV) by real-time RT-PCR. *Euro Surveill.* **2020**, *25*. [CrossRef] [PubMed]
13. Oostdijk, E.A.; De Jonge, E.; Kullberg, B.J.; Natsch, S.; De Smet, A.M.; Vandenbroucke-Grauls, C.M.J.E.; van der Vorm, E.; Bonten, M.J.M. SWAB-Richtlijn: Selectieve Decontaminatie bij Patiënten op de Intensive Care. 2018. Available online: https://swab.nl/nl/selectieve-decontaminatie-sdd (accessed on 22 May 2020).
14. Vergidis, P.; Moore, C.B.; Novak-Frazer, L.; Rautemaa-Richardson, R.; Walker, A.; Denning, D.W.; Richardson, M.D. High-volume culture and quantitative real-time PCR for the detection of *Aspergillus* in sputum. *Clin. Microbiol. Infect.* **2019**, in press. [CrossRef] [PubMed]
15. Ullmann, A.J.; Aguado, J.M.; Arikan-Akdagli, S.; Denning, D.W.; Groll, A.H.; Lagrou, K.; Lass-Flörl, C.; Lewis, R.E.; Munoz, P.; Verweij, P.E.; et al. Diagnosis and management of *Aspergillus* diseases: Executive summary of the 2017 ESCMID-ECMM-ERS guideline. *Clin. Microbiol. Infect.* **2018**, *24* (Suppl. 1), e1–e38. [CrossRef] [PubMed]
16. Chowdhary, A.; Kathuria, S.; Xu, J.P.; Meis, J.F. Emergence of azole-resistant *Aspergillus fumigatus* strains due to agricultural azole use creates an increasing threat to human health. *PLoS Pathog.* **2013**, *9*, e1003633. [CrossRef]
17. Talento, A.F.; Dunne, K.; Murphy, N.; O'Connell, B.; Chan, G.; Joyce, E.A.; Hagen, F.; Meis, J.F.; Fahy, R.; Bacon, L.; et al. Post-influenzal triazole-resistant aspergillosis following allogeneic stem cell transplantation. *Mycoses* **2018**, *61*, 570–575. [CrossRef]
18. Chowdhary, A.; Sharma, C.; Meis, J.F. Azole-resistant aspergillosis: Epidemiology, molecular mechanisms, and treatment. *J. Infect. Dis.* **2017**, *216*, S436–S444. [CrossRef]
19. Lestrade, P.P.; Meis, J.F.; Melchers, W.J.; Verweij, P.E. Triazole resistance in *Aspergillus fumigatus*: Recent insights and challenges for patient management. *Clin. Microbiol. Infect.* **2019**, *25*, 799–806. [CrossRef]

20. Ahmad, S.; Joseph, L.; Hagen, F.; Meis, J.F.; Khan, Z. Concomitant occurrence of itraconazole-resistant and -susceptible strains of *Aspergillus fumigatus* in routine cultures. *J. Antimicrob. Chemother.* **2015**, *70*, 412–415. [CrossRef]
21. Singh, A.; Sharma, B.; Kumar Mahto, K.; Meis, J.F.; Chowdhary, A. High-frequency direct detection of triazole resistance in *Aspergillus fumigatus* from patients with chronic pulmonary fungal diseases in India. *J. Fungi* **2020**, *6*, 67. [CrossRef]
22. Lestrade, P.P.; Buil, J.B.; van der Beek, M.T.; Kuijper, E.J.; van Dijk, K.; Kampinga, G.A.; Rijnders, B.J.A.; Vonk, A.G.; de Greeff, S.C.; Schoffelen, A.F.; et al. Paradoxal trends in azole-resistant *Aspergillus fumigatus* in a national multicenter surveillance program, 2013–2018. *Emerg. Infect. Dis.* **2020**, *26*. [CrossRef]
23. Blot, S.; Rello, J.; Koulenti, D. Diagnosing invasive pulmonary aspergillosis in ICU patients: Putting the puzzle together. *Curr. Opin. Crit. Care* **2019**, *25*, 430–437. [CrossRef] [PubMed]
24. Donnelly, J.P.; Chen, S.C.; Kauffman, C.A.; Steinbach, W.J.; Baddley, J.W.; Verweij, P.E.; Clancy, C.J.; Wingard, J.R.; Lockhart, S.R.; Groll, A.H.; et al. Revision and update of the consensus definitions of invasive fungal disease from the European Organization for Research and Treatment of Cancer and the Mycoses Study Group Education and Research Consortium. *Clin. Infect. Dis.* **2019**, in press. [CrossRef] [PubMed]
25. Blot, S.I.; Taccone, F.S.; Van den Abeele, A.M.; Bulpa, P.; Meersseman, W.; Brusselaers, N.; Dimopoulos, G.; Paiva, J.A.; Misset, B.; Rello, J.; et al. A clinical algorithm to diagnose invasive pulmonary aspergillosis in critically ill patients. *Am. J. Respir. Crit. Care Med.* **2012**, *186*, 56–64. [CrossRef]
26. Wahidi, M.M.; Lamb, C.; Murgu, S.; Musani, A.; Shojaee, S.; Sachdeva, A.; Maldonado, F.; Mahmood, K.; Kinsey, M.; Sethi, S.; et al. American Association for Bronchology and Interventional Pulmonology (AABIP) statement on the use of bronchoscopy and respiratory specimen collection in patients with suspected or confirmed COVID-19 infection. *J. Bronchol. Interv. Pulmonol.* **2020**. [CrossRef] [PubMed]
27. Meersseman, W.; Lagrou, K.; Maertens, J.; Wilmer, A.; Hermans, G.; Vanderschueren, S.; Spriet, I.; Verbeken, E.; Van Wijngaerden, E. Galactomannan in bronchoalveolar lavage fluid: A tool for diagnosing aspergillosis in intensive care unit patients. *Am. J. Respir. Crit. Care Med.* **2008**, *177*, 27–34. [CrossRef] [PubMed]
28. Verweij, P.E.; Weemaes, C.M.; Curfs, J.H.; Bretagne, S.; Meis, J.F. Failure to detect circulating Aspergillus markers in a patient with chronic granulomatous disease and invasive aspergillosis. *J. Clin. Microbiol.* **2000**, *38*, 3900–3901. [CrossRef]
29. Talento, A.F.; Dunne, K.; Joyce, E.A.; Palmer, M.; Johnson, E.; White, P.L.; Springer, J.; Loeffler, J.; Ryan, T.; Collins, D.; et al. A prospective study of fungal biomarkers to improve management of invasive fungal diseases in a mixed specialty critical care unit. *J. Crit. Care* **2017**, *40*, 119–127. [CrossRef]
30. Acosta, J.; Catalan, M.; del Palacio-Peréz-Medel, A.; Lora, D.; Montejo, J.C.; Cuetara, M.S.; Moragues, M.D.; Ponton, J.; del Palacio, A. A prospective comparison of galactomannan in bronchoalveolar lavage fluid for the diagnosis of pulmonary invasive aspergillosis in medical patients under intensive care: Comparison with the diagnostic performance of galactomannan and of (1→3)-β-d-glucan chromogenic assay in serum samples. *Clin. Microbiol. Infect.* **2011**, *17*, 1053–1060. [CrossRef]
31. Acosta, J.; Catalan, M.; Palacio-Pérez-Medel, A.; Montejo, J.; De-La-Cruz-Bértolo, J.; Moragues, M.; Pontón, J.; Finkelman, M.; Palacio, A. Prospective study in critically ill non-neutropenic patients: Diagnostic potential of (1,3)-β-D-glucan assay and circulating galactomannan for the diagnosis of invasive fungal disease. *Eur. J. Clin. Microbiol. Infect. Dis.* **2011**, *31*, 721–731. [CrossRef]
32. Boch, T.; Reinwald, M.; Spiess, B.; Liebregts, T.; Schellongowski, P.; Meybohm, P.; Rath, P.M.; Steinmann, J.; Trinkmann, F.; Britsch, S.; et al. Detection of invasive pulmonary aspergillosis in critically ill patients by combined use of conventional culture, galactomannan, 1,3-β-D-glucan and *Aspergillus* specific nested polymerase chain reaction in a prospective pilot study. *J. Crit. Care* **2018**, *47*, 198–203. [CrossRef] [PubMed]
33. De Vlieger, G.; Lagrou, K.; Maertens, J.; Verbeken, E.; Meersseman, W.; Van Wijngaerden, E. Beta-D-glucan detection as a diagnostic test for invasive aspergillosis in immunocompromised critically ill patients with symptoms of respiratory infection: An autopsy-based study. *J. Clin. Microbiol.* **2011**, *49*, 3783–3787. [CrossRef] [PubMed]
34. Lahmer, T.; Neuenhahn, M.; Held, J.; Rasch, S.; Schmid, R.M.; Huber, W. Comparison of 1,3-β-d-glucan with galactomannan in serum and bronchoalveolar fluid for the detection of *Aspergillus* species in immunosuppressed mechanical ventilated critically ill patients. *J. Crit. Care* **2016**, *36*, 259–264. [CrossRef] [PubMed]

35. Vanderbeke, L.; Van Wijngaerden, E.; Maertens, J.; Wauters, J.; Lagrou, K. Diagnosis of invasive aspergillosis in intensive care unit patients. *Curr. Fungal Infect. Rep.* **2020**. [CrossRef]
36. Johnson, G.L.; Sarker, S.-J.; Nannini, F.; Ferrini, A.; Taylor, E.; Lass-Flörl, C.; Mutschlechner, W.; Bustin, S.A.; Agrawal, S.G. *Aspergillus*-specific lateral-flow device and real-time PCR testing of bronchoalveolar lavage fluid: A combination biomarker approach for clinical diagnosis of invasive pulmonary aspergillosis. *J. Clin. Microbiol.* **2015**, *53*, 2103–2108. [CrossRef] [PubMed]
37. Hoenigl, M.; Prattes, J.; Spiess, B.; Wagner, J.; Prueller, F.; Raggam, R.B.; Posch, V.; Duettmann, W.; Hoenigl, K.; Wölfler, A.; et al. Performance of galactomannan, 1,3-β-d-glucan, *Aspergillus* lateral-flow device, conventional culture, and PCR tests with bronchoalveolar lavage fluid for diagnosis of invasive pulmonary aspergillosis. *J. Clin. Microbiol.* **2014**, *52*, 2039–2045. [CrossRef]
38. Jenks, J.D.; Mehta, S.R.; Taplitz, R.; Aslam, S.; Reed, S.L.; Hoenigl, M. Point-of-care diagnosis of invasive aspergillosis in non-neutropenic patients: *Aspergillus* galactomannan lateral flow assay versus *Aspergillus*-specific lateral flow device test in bronchoalveolar lavage. *Mycoses* **2019**, *62*, 230–236. [CrossRef]
39. Eigl, S.; Prattes, J.; Lackner, M.; Willinger, B.; Spiess, B.; Reinwald, M.; Selitsch, B.; Meilinger, M.; Neumeister, P.; Reischies, F.; et al. Multicenter evaluation of a lateral-flow device test for diagnosing invasive pulmonary aspergillosis in ICU patients. *Crit. Care* **2015**, *19*, 178. [CrossRef]

Journal of *Fungi*

MDPI

Review

COVID-19-Associated Candidiasis (CAC): An Underestimated Complication in the Absence of Immunological Predispositions?

Amir Arastehfar [1,*,†], Agostinho Carvalho [2,3,*,†], M. Hong Nguyen [4], Mohammad Taghi Hedayati [5], Mihai G. Netea [6,7,8], David S. Perlin [1] and Martin Hoenigl [9,10,11,*]

1 Center for Discovery and Innovation, Hackensack Meridian Health, Nutley, NJ 07110, USA; david.perlin@hmh-cdi.org
2 Life and Health Sciences Research Institute (ICVS), School of Medicine, University of Minho, 4710-057 Braga, Portugal
3 ICVS/3B's—PT Government Associate Laboratory, 4710-057 Guimarães/Braga, Portugal
4 Department of Medicine, University of Pittsburgh, Pittsburgh, PA 15261, USA; mhn5@pitt.edu
5 Invasive Fungi Research Center, Department of Medical Mycology, School of Medicine, Mazandaran University of Medical Sciences, Sari 4815733971, Iran; hedayatimt@gmail.com
6 Department of Internal Medicine and Radboud Center for Infectious Diseases, Radboud University Medical Centre, 6500HB Nijmegen, The Netherlands; Mihai.Netea@radboudumc.nl
7 Department of Genomics & Immunoregulation, Life and Medical Sciences Institute, University of Bonn, 53115 Bonn, Germany
8 Radboud Institute for Molecular Life Sciences, Radboud University Medical Center, 6525 GA Nijmegen, The Netherlands
9 Clinical and Translational Fungal-Working Group, University of California San Diego, La Jolla, CA 92093, USA
10 Section of Infectious Diseases and Tropical Medicine, Department of Internal Medicine, Medical University of Graz, 8036 Graz, Austria
11 Division of Infectious Diseases and Global Public Health, Department of Medicine, University of California, San Diego, San Diego, CA 92093, USA
* Correspondence: a.arastehfar.nl@gmail.com (A.A.); agostinhocarvalho@med.uminho.pt (A.C.); hoeniglmartin@gmail.com (M.H.);
Tel./Fax: +1-201-880-3100 (A.A.); +351-253-604811 (A.C.); +1-619-543-5605 (M.H.)
† These authors contributed equally to this work.

Received: 11 September 2020; Accepted: 6 October 2020; Published: 8 October 2020

Abstract: The recent global pandemic of COVID-19 has predisposed a relatively high number of patients to acute respiratory distress syndrome (ARDS), which carries a risk of developing super-infections. *Candida* species are major constituents of the human mycobiome and the main cause of invasive fungal infections, with a high mortality rate. Invasive yeast infections (IYIs) are increasingly recognized as s complication of severe COVID-19. Despite the marked immune dysregulation in COVID-19, no prominent defects have been reported in immune cells that are critically required for immunity to *Candida*. This suggests that relevant clinical factors, including prolonged ICU stays, central venous catheters, and broad-spectrum antibiotic use, may be key factors causing COVID-19 patients to develop IYIs. Although data on the comparative performance of diagnostic tools are often lacking in COVID-19 patients, a combination of serological and molecular techniques may present a promising option for the identification of IYIs. Clinical awareness and screening are needed, as IYIs are difficult to diagnose, particularly in the setting of severe COVID-19. Echinocandins and azoles are the primary antifungal used to treat IYIs, yet the therapeutic failures exerted by multidrug-resistant *Candida* spp. such as *C. auris* and *C. glabrata* call for the development of new antifungal drugs with novel mechanisms of action.

Keywords: candidemia; candiduria; oral candidiasis; mycobiome

1. Introduction

Yeast species belonging to the *Candida* genus, including *Candida albicans*, *Candida glabrata*, *Candida parapsilosis*, *Candida tropicalis*, and *Candida krusei*, are the most prevalent fungal species inhabiting various mucosal surfaces, such as the skin and the respiratory, digestive, and urinary tracts [1,2]. Although being commensal within the human host, *Candida* species are equipped with virulence attributes, enabling them to invade when opportunities arise and cause various infections in humans, especially when the immune system is impaired [2]. Superficial infections, such as skin disorders; mucosal infections, including oropharyngeal or vulvovaginitis candidiasis; and invasive candidiasis are established clinical entities of candidiasis [3–8]. *Candida* is among the most frequently recovered pathogen in the intensive care unit (ICU), affecting between 6% and 10% of patients, and some studies have noted an increasing trend for candidemia [9]. The estimated mortality attributed to invasive candidiasis is 19–40% [10]. This mortality is even higher among ICU patients, approaching 70% [11]. Apart from being associated with excess economic costs and approximately 1.5 million annual deaths [8], the new landscape of candidemia reveals an increasing incidence of non-*albicans Candida* (NAC) species, with intrinsic resistance to antifungals and/or with a propensity to rapidly acquire antifungal resistance [12]. More troubling is the recent emergence of multidrug-resistant (MDR) *Candida* species, including *C. glabrata* and *C. auris* [13–16], the increasing trend of fluconazole-resistant *C. parapsilosis* and *C. tropicalis* [13,17], and inherently resistant *C. krusei*, which notoriously affect the efficacy of antifungal treatment.

The recent global pandemic of COVID-19 has resulted in an unprecedented 890,000 deaths worldwide [18]. A notable proportion of COVID-19 critically ill patients develop acute respiratory distress syndrome (ARDS), requiring intensive care unit (ICU) admission and mechanical ventilation, which in turn predisposes them to nosocomial infections due to bacterial and fungal infections [19,20]. Understanding the burden of COVID-19 patients with secondary infections and their etiologic agents is paramount for the optimal management of COVID-19 patients. This knowledge will help to refine empiric antimicrobial management for patients with COVID-19 with the hope to improve patient outcomes.

Despite the recognition that airborne *Aspergillus fumigatus* is increasingly recognized as an important cause of fungal super-infections among critically ill COVID-19 patients [19], the incidence of candidiasis has not been evaluated in this context. Indeed, the wide use of antibiotics, corticosteroids, and central venous catheters, along with the damage exerted by SARS CoV-2 among patients with ARDS [19], may allow commensal *Candida* to cells to invade internal organs [20–27]. The goals of this manuscript are to review our current knowledge on *Candida* super-infections among COVID-19 patients, discuss the potential immunological and clinical factors predisposing these patients to invasive candidiasis, and outline what studies are needed to better define the epidemiology of this superinfection.

2. Immunology

2.1. General Pathophysiology of SARS COV-2

Similar to other SARS coronaviruses, the pathophysiology of SARS-CoV-2 involves targeting and invading epithelial cells and type II pneumocytes through the binding of the SARS spike protein to the angiotensin-converting enzyme 2 (ACE2) receptor [28]. During the course of the host–virus interaction, the type 2 transmembrane protease TMPRSS2 cleaves the S1/S2 domain of the viral spike protein [29] and promotes viral entry into the target cells. ACE2 is required for protection from severe acute lung injury in ARDS [30], and the viral-mediated manipulation of this receptor is considered one major mechanism contributing to severe lung injury in selected COVID-19 patients. The degree of variability in the severity of disease is also supported, at least in part, by the existence of genetic variants that affect the ACE2 activity and underlie an increased susceptibility to ARDS and worse prognosis [31].

Besides the implications of ACE2 in the pathogenesis of COVID-19, recent studies have also suggested that the disruption of the renin-angiotensin system and/or the kallikrein-kinin system could contribute to the detrimental inflammatory phenotype observed in patients with severe COVID-19 [32,33].

2.2. *Does Immunity Renders Susceptibility to Invasive Yeast Infections?*

Infection with SARS-CoV2 elicits an immune response that triggers an inflammatory cascade as the result of the activity of innate immune cells. However, the dynamics of how the immune system senses and responds to SARS-CoV-2 is just unfolding, which limits our understanding of possible immune-mediated pathways contributing to the pathogenesis COVID-19-associated candidiasis (CAC). Cell types important for host defense against *Candida*, such as neutrophils and monocytes/macrophages, are not affected by SARS-CoV-2, suggesting that they are not responsible for CAC. Indeed, single-cell analyses of bronchoalveolar lavages from critically ill patients with COVID-19 showed an abundance of monocyte-derived macrophages [34]. Similarly, an increased peripheral neutrophil-to-lymphocyte ratio was also observed in severe cases of COVID-19, and was likely associated with unfavorable prognosis [35]. While the increasing numbers (and activation profiles) of these cells may contribute to tissue damage and the severity of disease, they are an unlikely risk factor for invasive candidiasis. One exception is the decreased expression of human leukocyte antigen DR on the membrane of circulating monocytes [36], which is considered a marker of immune paralysis; however, its relevance in susceptibility to candidemia is unclear. The clear immune defect in patients with COVID-19 is, on the other hand, lymphopenia; however, an isolated decrease in lymphocyte numbers, as also experienced by HIV patients, is not associated with an increase in susceptibility to systemic *Candida* infections. Taken together, these findings support the concept that classical risk factors for invasive candidiasis, rather than an overt immune dysfunction, are the major drivers of susceptibility to CAC.

3. Epidemiology of CAC, Clinical and Microbiological Factors: Current Paradigm

To obtain studies reporting yeast infections among patients with COVID-19, we included all studies published up to September 10, 2020. Our search included yeast, *Candida*, COVID-19, fungal super-infection +COVID-19, and fungal super-infections + COVID-19, and we used both the Google and PubMed search engines. The extent of CAC (both superficial and invasive) varies by country and region. Studies from Spain [37], India [27], Iran [22], Italy [26], the UK [23], and China [20] have reported rates of 0.7% (7/989), 2.5% (15/596), 5% (53/ 1059), 8% (3/43), 12.6% (17/135), and 23.5% (4/17) [20], respectively (Table 1). Although a previous study from Iran indicated a relatively low level of oral candidiasis (OC) among patients with COVID-19 (53/1059), apparently that study included all the patients who presented with COVID-19 but not those developing ARDS, which may have resulted in an underestimation of OC in the context of COVID-19 [22].

Table 1. Clinical and microbiological features of COVID-19-associated invasive yeast infections in studies with detailed clinical and microbiological data.

Country (Case Number; %) [ref.]	Age/Sex	Underlying Conditions	Risk Factors	Hospitalization Duration	Days to Camdidemia Positivity	Species (Resistance Pattern)	Treatment	Outcome
India (15/596; 2.5%) [27]	25/F	CLD with grade II encephalopathy, AKD	Antibiotic use, CVC, and UC	35	14	*C. auris* (MAR), blood culture	AMB	Survived
	52/M	HT, DM	Antibiotic use, steroid therapy, CVC, and UC	20	14 and 17	*C. auris* (FLCR), blood culture	MFG and AMB	Died
	82/F	HT, DM, hypothoidism, on dialysis for CKD stage 5	Antibiotic use, steroid therapy, CVC, and UC	60	42 and 47	*C. auris* (FLCR), blood culture	MFG	Died
	86/F	CLD, IHD, DM	Antibiotic use, steroid therapy, CVC, and UC	21	10	*C. auris* (FLCR), blood culture	MFG	Died
	66/M	HT, DM, asthma	Antibiotic use, CVC, and UC	20	11 and 15	*C. auris* (FLCR+AMBR), blood culture	MFG and AMB	Survived
	71/M	Hypothoidism, on dialysis for CKD stage 5	Antibiotic use, steroid therapy, CVC, and UC	32	12 and 17	*C. auris* (FLCR), blood culture	MFG	Died
	67/M	HT, DM, COPD	Antibiotic use, steroid therapy, CVC, and UC	21	11	*C. auris* (FLCR+AMBR), blood culture	AMB and MFG	Survived
	72/M	HT, CLD	Antibiotic use, steroid therapy, CVC, and UC	27	16 and 19	*C. auris* (MAR+AMBR), blood culture	MFG	Died
	81/M	DM, HT, IHD	Antibiotic use, steroid therapy, CVC, and UC	20	15	*C. auris* (MAR), blood culture	MFG	Died
	69/M	HT, asthma	Antibiotic use, steroid therapy, CVC, and UC	21	14	*C. auris* (FLCR+AMBR), blood culture	MFG	Survived
	56/M	HT, COPD	Antibiotic use, CVC, and UC	18	7	*C. tropicalis* (S), blood culture	MFG	Survived
	69/M	HT, DM, obesity, IHD	Antibiotic use, CVC, and UC	27	8	*C. albicans* (S), blood culture	MFG	Survived
	43/F	HT	Antibiotic use, steroid therapy, CVC, and UC	24	12	*C. albicans* (S), blood culture	MFG	Survived
	47/M	Asthma, DM	Antibiotic use, CVC, and UC	18	5	*C. albicans* (S), blood culture	AMB and MFG	Died
	66/M	HT	Antibiotic use, steroid therapy, CVC, and UC	28	7	*C. krusei* (IFR), blood culture	AMB	Died
Oman (5/ ND) [A] [25]	76/M	None	Antibiotic use, CVC	ND	ND	*C. albicans* (S), CVC culture	No	Died
	68/M	HT	Antibiotic use, CVC	ND	ND	*C. albicans* (S), blood culture	CAS + CVC removal	Died
	38/M	HT, dyslipidemia, old stroke	Antibiotic use, CVC	ND	ND	*C. glabrata* (S), blood culture	MFG→CAS→AMB	Died
	64/M	HT	Antibiotic use, CVC	ND	ND	*C. albicans* + *C. tropicalis* (S), blood culture	CAS+VRC	Survived
	49/M	None	Antibiotic use, CVC	ND	ND	*C. albicans* (S), blood culture	CAS	Survived

Table 1. *Cont.*

Country (Case Number; %) [ref.]	Age/Sex	Underlying Conditions	Risk Factors	Hospitalization Duration	Days to Camdidemia Positivity	Species (Resistance Pattern)	Treatment	Outcome
UK (17/135; 12.6%) [23]	ND	HT, obesity	CVC	ND	ND	No ID, CVC	FLC	Died
	ND	HT		ND	ND	*Rhodotorula* spp., blood culture	CAS, LAMB	Died
	ND	Oseophagectomy, cancer	Hydrocortisone	ND	ND	No ID, from chest drain	FLC	Died
	ND	Ulcerative colitis	CVC	ND	ND	*C. albicans*, CVC	None	Survived
	ND	DM, HT, obesity, asthma	CVC	ND	ND	*C. albicans*, CVC	FLC	Survived
	ND	HT, asthma		ND	ND	*C. albicans*, blood culture, BDG = 156, 95, 86, *Candida* PCR = Positive	CAS	Survived
	ND	Haem, cardiac		ND	ND	*C. albicans*, blood culture	None	Died
	ND	None	CVC	ND	ND	*C. albicans*, CVC	FLC	Survived
	ND	Cardiac, CKD, cancer	CVC	ND	ND	*C. albicans*, CVC	CAS	Died
	ND	Asthma, inflammatory, irritable bowel syndrome	CVC	ND	ND	*C. albicans*, CVC	VRC	Died
	ND	None	CVC	ND	ND	*C. parapsilosis*, CVC	CAS	Survived
	ND	None	CVC	ND	ND	*C. albicans*, CVC and blood culture	FLC	Died
	ND	None		ND	ND	*C. albicans*, blood culture, BDG > 500, *Candida* PCR = Positive	FLC, CAS	Survived
	ND	DM, HT, Obesity	CVC	ND	ND	*C. albicans*, CVC	FLC	Survived
	ND	Hepatitis, intravenous drug user, neutropenia, cellulitis		ND	ND	*C. albicans* + *C. parapsilosis*, blood culture, BDG = 386	FLC, LAMB	Survived
	ND	DM, inflammatory, alcoholic	Steroid therapy (ND)	ND	ND	*C. albicans*, ascites culture	CAS, VRC	Survived
	ND	DM, HT		ND	ND	*C. albicans*, CVC, BDG > 500	FLC, VRC	Died
Italy (3/43; 8%) [26]	67/M	Cerebral ischemia	Parentral nutrition, antibiotic use, CVC, and Tocilizumab (8 mg/kg)	ND	13	*C. albicans*, blood culture	CAS+FLC	Survived
	58/M	HT	Parenteral nutrition and Tocilizumab (8 mg/kg)	ND	17	*C. tropicalis*, blood culture	CAS	Survived
	78/M	DM and obesity	Parenteral nutrition, antibiotic use, steroid therapy, CVC, and Tocilizumab (8 mg/kg)	ND	13	*C. parapsilosis*, blood culture	CAS+FLC	Survived
Italy (1/ND) [24]	79/M	DM, IHD, stadium IV peripheral artery disease	Antibiotic use and surgery	35	53	*C. glabrata* (PER), blood culture	CAS	Died
Greece (2/ND) [21]	76/M	HT	Antibiotic use, Ultra-Levure (250–500 mg/day)	80	35 (4 days after Ultra-Levure)	*S. cerevisiae* (S), blood culture	AND→FLC	Survived
	73/M	HT and DM	Antibiotic use, Ultra-Levure (250–500 mg/day)	Transferred to a regional hospital	15 (6 days after Ultra-Levure)	*S. cerevisiae* (S), blood culture	AND→FLC	Survived

A. The total number of severely ill patients was not determined for studies from Italy [24], Greece [21], and Oman [25]. AKD: Acute kidney disease; CKD: Chronic kidney disease; CLD: Chronic liver disease; COPD: Chronic obstructive pulmonary disease; DM: Diabetes mellitus; HT: Hypertension; IHD: Ischemic heart diseases; CVC: Central venous catheter; UC: Urinary catheter; AMB: Amphotericin B; LAMB: Liposomal AMB; MFG: Micafungin; CAS: Caspofungin; VRC: Voriconazole; FLC: Fluconazole; S: Susceptible; FLCR: Fluconazole-resistant; AMBR: Amphotericin B-resistant; IFR: Intrinsically fluconazole-resistant MAR: Multiazole-resistant; MDR: Multidrug-resistant; PER: Pan-echinocandin-resistant; ND: Not determined; PCR: Polymerase chain reaction; BDG: Beta-d-glucan.

A study from Spain reported a rate of 0.7% (7/989) of fungal super-infections complicating hospitalized COVID-19 patients: four were caused by molds and three by *Candida* (one each of candidemia, candiduria, and complicated intraabdominal candidiasis (IAC)) [37]. Similarly, a recent study from the UK reported a similar prevalence of invasive yeast infections and invasive pulmonary aspergillosis (12.6% vs. 14.1%) among COVID-19 patients who presented with ARDS [23]. A study from Greece reported that two COVID-19 patients residing in an ICU developed bloodstream infection due to *Saccharomyces cerevisiae* a few days (4–6 days) after receiving a probiotic supplement (Ultra-Levure) which contains this yeast. Interestingly, none of the 320 patients admitted to the same unit in the previous 4 years developed *S. cerevisiae* fungemia while receiving the same probiotic [21]. This observation, while anecdotal, suggests that the sepsis syndrome or septic shock associated with severe COVID-19 may damage the intestinal mucosal barrier, enabling the translocation of concentrated fungus in probiotics (250–500 mg/day in this case), leading to fungemia [38,39]. This study cautions about the routine use of prophylactic probiotics among critically ill COVID-19 cases in the ICU setting.

Moreover, a recent study from Italy also reported three candidemia cases among critically ill COVID-19 patients following treatment with tocilizumab, an IL-6 receptor monoclonal blocking agent [26]. Central venous catheterization (CVC) (32/43; 74.5%), antibiotics (26/43; 60.5%), and steroid therapy use (13/43; 13.2%) were among the most prominent risk factors reported (Table 1). Overall, the mortality rate of invasive *Candida* infections was approximately 46% (20/ 43), which varied depending on the species and the antifungal used to treat invasive yeast infections. Indeed, this mortality rate is presumably higher than that of severely ill patients with COVID-19, ranging between 25.8% [40] and 30.9% [41]. Per species, the mortality rate was the highest for patients infected with *C. glabrata* (2/2; 100%), *C. auris* (6/10; 60%), and *C. albicans* (8/19; 42%), while those treated with *C. tropicalis*, *C. parapsilosis*, and multiple *Candida* species all survived (two patients infected with *C. krusei* and *Rhodotorula* spp. and two with unknown species also died). It is noteworthy that those results may be misleading due to the limited numbers, since *C. tropicalis* has been shown before to be associated with the poorest prognosis and also carries a high rate of mortality when compared to other non-*Candida albicans Candida* species [42,43].

According to recent studies detailing invasive yeast infections among critically ill COVID-19 patients (21, 23–27), *C. albicans* (19/43; 44.1%) was shown to be the most prevalent yeast species, followed by *C. auris* (10/43; 23.2%); *C. glabrata*, *C. parapsilosis*, *C. tropicalis*, and *S. cerevisiae* (2/43; 4.6% each); and *C. krusei* and *Rhodotorula* spp. (1/43; 2.3% each). Of note, there was no species identity reported for two yeast isolates obtained from catheter and chest drain, and two patients had mixed invasive yeast infections caused by *C. albicans* + *C. parapsilosis* and *C. albicans* + *C. tropicalis* (Table 1). Importantly, *C. auris* was the most prevalent *Candida* species from the Indian study, while *C. albicans* was the most prevalent in the other studies. Where antifungal susceptibility testing was performed, the resistance patterns varied depending on the species. For instance, resistance to fluconazole, multiple azoles (fluconazole and voriconazole), and multidrugs (fluconazole and AMB) was noted for 100%, 30%, and 40% of the *C. auris* isolates, respectively, and only one *C. glabrata* isolate was echinocandin-resistant (Table 1). Persistent invasive yeast infections have been noted during the course of antifungal therapy, while the yeasts isolated showed susceptible profiles to the antifungal used for treatment [25,27]. Most notably, 67% of the patients who died with invasive yeast infections due to *C. auris* showed persistent candidemia, despite being treated with micafungin [27] in the absence of resistance, which might be explained by other host and pathogen-related factors [44–46]. Therefore, these data highlight the urgency of conducting comprehensive studies elucidating the real burden of each entity among COVID-19 cases manifesting ARDS.

4. Risk Factors

The risk factors for CAC can be divided into two groups. The first group includes common risk factors predisposing ICU patients to invasive candidiasis. These include diabetes mellitus, renal failure requiring hemodialysis, abdominal surgery, triple lumen catheters, parenteral nutrition, receipt of multiple antibiotics, length of ICU stay >7 days, and prior abdominal infections [10,47,48]. Additionally, indwelling central venous catheters are widely used among COVID-19 patients residing in ICUs [49]. Indeed, catheters are historically known as a portal of entry for acquiring nosocomial *Candida* infections, such as *Candida auris* and *C. parapsilosis* [15,16,50,51]. Of note, approximately 82% of CVC-recovered yeast isolates were *C. albicans* (9/ 11) (Table 1), which also shows that other *Candida* species have the potential to cause CVC-related invasive yeast infections. Unlike endogenously acquired *Candida* species, such as *C. glabrata*, that require previous exposure to antifungals drugs to become drug-resistant, drug-resistant *C. auris* and *C. parapsilosis* can persist on the hospital environments, devices, and hands of healthcare workers and subsequently cause drug-resistant candidiasis and/or candidemia among antifungal-naïve patients [15–17,50–53]. It is also noteworthy that some studies have found an association between antibiotic use and the emergence of candidemia due to *Candida* species exhibiting a high minimum inhibitory concentration (MIC) and/or intrinsic resistance to fluconazole [54,55]. Furthermore, the development of invasive candidiasis is often preceded by the *Candida* colonization of the skin and mucous membrane. *Candida* colonization at multiple body sites is a strong predictor of invasive candidiasis [56]. Along the same line, the *Candida* colonization of the airway has been observed in 20% of patients after 48 h of being on mechanical ventilation, and the longer the duration of ventilation, the higher the colonization rate [3]. Up to 94% of hospitalized patients with COVID-19 receive antimicrobial agents [57–59], and this might further heighten the *Candida* colonization rate. Patients with sepsis or septic shock, commonly observed in severe COVID-19 patients in the ICU, may develop a leaky gut that facilitates *Candida* translocation from the GI tract into systemic circulation [39,60–62].

The second group of risk factors are more specifically associated with COVID-19. First, patients with severe respiratory failure associated with COVID-19 might require extracorporeal membrane oxygenation (ECMO) [63]. ECMO involves a higher number of vascular catheters (pulmonary and peripheral arterial catheters and ECMO cannula in addition to central venous catheters). ECMO is also associated with a clotting tendency that facilitates microbial pathogen (bacteria and fungus) adhesion to the catheters, as well as leukopenia that results from the sequestration of leukocytes in the lung capillaries and peripheral tissues, and adhesion to and lysis of leukocytes by ECMO circuit. ECMO cannula are often colonized by skin commensals such as *Candida* and coagulase-negative *Staphylococcus*, a condition that predisposes one to bloodstream infection. Altogether, these risk factors predispose one to systemic infection. Second, corticosteroids have been increasingly used among hospitalized patients with COVID-19 [19]. Corticosteroids have immunosuppressive effects on neutrophils, monocytesm and macrophages and predispose patients to invasive candidiasis. Lastly, whether the severe lung epithelium damage exerted by SARS CoV-2 facilitates *Candida* adherence to basement membrane causing subsequent invasive pulmonary candidiasis is not known. To date, primary *Candida* pneumonitis is considered to be rare.

5. Diagnosis

The diagnosis of candidemia and other forms of invasive candidiasis remains challenging, which is mostly due to the low number of yeast cells in circulation or infected tissue [64], a requirement of an invasive procedure for diagnosing deep-seated candidiasis, and the use of non-fungal-specific media to culture clinical samples [65]. While culture remains the gold standard, approximately 50% of the invasive candidiasis are not identified by blood culture, and the application of non-culture diagnostics—i.e., β-D-Glucan (BDG) and mannan antigen testing, and molecular platforms such as PCR and T2 Candida panel—are recommended to improve the diagnosis [64]. BDG (Associates of Cape Cod Diagnostics; MA, USA) is a panfungal marker and therefore a positive result is not specific for invasive candidiasis. The sensitivity and specificity for diagnosing invasive candidiasis are around 80% [66,67], and can further be increased when combined with procalcitonin, which may help to differentiate fungal from bacterial infections [68], but false positive results have been described, in particular in conditions associated with fungal translocation in the gut, such as sepsis or advanced liver cirrhosis [61,69]. BDG results should therefore be carefully evaluated and always interpreted with other clinical data. Importantly, serum BDG has been shown to be a reliable tool for antifungal stewardship, and has a high negative predictive value for invasive *Candida* infections, allowing for the early discontinuation of empirical antifungal therapy if tested from samples drawn before treatment initiation [70,71]. Enzyme-linked immunosorbent assay (ELISA) kits for the detection of *Candida* mannan antigen are commercially available to detect *Candida* in serum samples for the diagnosis of invasive candidiasis (Platelia™ Candida Ag, Bio-Rad), and are associated with a relatively high specificity and sensitivity [72]. In a recent meta-analysis, blood PCR was associated with a pooled sensitivity and specificity for proven or probable invasive candidiasis vs. at-risk controls of 95% and 92%, respectively [73]. The recently developed T2Candida Panel (T2Biosystems) combines ITS2 region amplification and T2 magnetic resonance, and can directly detect *Candida* spp. in EDTA blood samples within 5 h and has proved efficient for the diagnosis of candidemia and intra-abdominal candidiasis, although the technical demands can be a drawback [74–76].

Combining multiple techniques is recommended in order to improve the sensitivity of the techniques [64,77,78]. However, while serum BDG testing and screening has been used successfully in COVID-19 patients for the detection of COVID associated aspergillosis [19], the utility of other techniques remains to be determined in the context of COVID-19 patients with ARDS.

6. Treatment and Future Directions

Since invasive yeast infections are associated with a higher mortality in COVID-19 cases not receiving antifungal treatment compared to those receiving it [23], prompt diagnosis and treatment is of paramount importance to achieve clinical success. The management of invasive candidiasis in patients with COVID-19 is similar to that of non-COVID-19 patients. Echinocandins are the treatment of choice for invasive *Candida* infections, with fluconazole, liposomal amphotericin B, voriconazole, posaconazolem and isavuconazole being the second line alternatives [79–81]. Source control, including, if feasible, the removal of central venous catheters in candidemic patients, is a major determinant factor of the outcome. Echinocandins are usually well tolerated and have a favorable pharmacokinetic (PK) profile, with very few drug–drug interactions [82]. A major drawback of echinocandins is their intravenous formulation. While not impacting most hospitalized and ICU patients, it is a factor for step-down therapy or prophylaxis. The triterpenoid ibrexafungerp is a new class of structurally distinct glucan synthase inhibitors, which is currently being evaluated in various phase III trials, showing an excellent bioavailability after oral intake [83]. Moreover, the penetration of currently available echinocandins into the abdominal infection site might not be optimal, and the emergence of echinocandin-resistant *Candida* isolates during treatment, especially *C. glabrata*, is problematic [44,84]. The newer generation of echinocandins, such as the long PK and the once-weekly drug rezafungin, have shown a favorable penetration in models of IAC when compared to other echinocandins [84]. Another novel antifungal in the pipeline that will likely advance the management of invasive candida infections in the near future is fosmanogepix. It has a novel mechanism of action that inhibits the highly conserved fungal enzyme Gwt1, which is essential for the biosynthesis of glycosylphosphatidylinositol anchors.

Among patients with septic shock attributed to invasive candidiasis, the timely administration of antifungal therapy is paramount for a favorable outcome. Consistent with the data described in this overview, we need to increase our efforts to understand the full extent of this invasive fungal complication in COVID-19, and to design the best diagnosis and therapy. What should be done in the future? Since blood culture has a poor sensitivity and delayed turnaround time, the development of predictive scores or diagnostic tests that yield high positive and/ or negative predictive values is sorely needed. Diagnostics directly from blood may offer the fastest laboratory results for high-risk patients. Among COVID-19 patients, the incidence of super-infections due to *Candida* is currently not known. It is also unknown whether *Candida* super-infection leads to excess mortality or if it is merely a marker of the severity of COVID-19 infection. Well-designed and careful epidemiologic studies are needed to define the true burden of invasive candidiasis among patients with COVID-19. Prospective studies that include systematic blood and other biological sample collection might enhance future research in invasive *Candida* infections.

Author Contributions: Conceptualization, M.H., A.A., and A.C.; writing—original draft preparation, A.A., A.C., M.H., M.H.N., M.T.H., D.S.P., M.G.N; writing—review and editing, A.A., A.C., M.H., M.H.N., M.T.H., D.S.P., M.G.N. All authors have read and agreed to the published version of the manuscript.

Funding: This research received no external funding.

Acknowledgments: We thank Farnaz Daneshnia for for revising the text.

Conflicts of Interest: M.H. received research funding by Gilead and Pfizer. D.S.P. receives research support and/or serves on advisory boards for Amplyx, Cidara, Scynexis, N8 Medical, Merck, Regeneron, and Pfizer. He also has a patent covering the detection of fungal species and drug resistance, as well as a pending patent on COVID-19 detection licensed to T2 Biosystems. A.C. was supported by the Fundação para a Ciência e a Tecnologia (FCT) (CEECIND/03628/2017 and PTDC/MED-GEN/28778/2017). Additional support was provided by FCT (UIDB/50026/2020 and UIDP/50026/2020), the Northern Portugal Regional Operational Programme (NORTE 2020), under the Portugal 2020 Partnership Agreement through the European Regional Development Fund (ERDF) (NORTE-01-0145-FEDER-000013 and NORTE-01-0145-FEDER-000023), the European Union's Horizon 2020 research and innovation program under grant agreement no. 847507, and the "la Caixa" Foundation (ID 100010434) and FCT under the agreement LCF/PR/HP17/52190003.

References

1. Hallen-Adams, H.E.; Suhr, M.J. Fungi in the healthy human gastrointestinal tract. *Virulence* **2017**, *8*, 352–358. [CrossRef] [PubMed]
2. Rolling, T.; Hohl, T.M.; Zhai, B. Minority report: The intestinal mycobiota in systemic infections. *Curr. Opin. Microbiol.* **2020**, *56*, 1–6. [CrossRef] [PubMed]
3. Azoulay, E.; Timsit, J.-F.; Tafflet, M.; De Lassence, A.; Darmon, M.; Zahar, J.-R.; Adrie, C.; Garrouste-Orgeas, M.; Cohen, Y.; Mourvillier, B.; et al. Candida Colonization of the Respiratory Tract and Subsequent Pseudomonas Ventilator-Associated Pneumonia. *Chest* **2006**, *129*, 110–117. [CrossRef] [PubMed]
4. Haron, E.; Vartivarian, S.; Anaissie, E.; Dekmezian, R.; Bodey, G.P. Primary Candida pneumonia. Experience at a large cancer center and review of the literature. *Medicine (Baltim.)* **1993**, *72*, 137–142. [CrossRef]
5. El-Ebiary, M.; Torres, A.; Fàbregas, N.; de la Bellacasa, J.P.; González, J.; Ramirez, J.; del Baño, D.; Hernández, C.; de Anta, M.T.J. Significance of the isolation of Candida species from respiratory samples in critically ill, non-neutropenic patients. An immediate postmortem histologic study. *Am. J. Respir. Crit. Care Med.* **1997**, *156*, 583–590. [CrossRef]
6. Meersseman, W.; Lagrou, K.; Spriet, I.; Maertens, J.; Verbeken, E.; Peetermans, W.E.; Van Wijngaerden, E. Significance of the isolation of Candida species from airway samples in critically ill patients: A prospective, autopsy study. *Intensive Care Med.* **2009**, *35*, 1526–1531. [CrossRef]
7. Schnabel, R.M.; Linssen, C.F.; Guion, N.; Van Mook, W.N.; Bergmans, D.C. Candida Pneumonia in Intensive Care Unit? *Open Forum Infect. Dis.* **2014**, *1*, ofu026. [CrossRef]
8. Brown, G.D.; Denning, D.W.; Gow, N.A.R.; Levitz, S.M.; Netea, M.G.; White, T.C. Hidden Killers: Human Fungal Infections. *Sci. Transl. Med.* **2012**, *4*, 165rv13. [CrossRef]
9. Lortholary, O.; The French Mycosis Study Group; Renaudat, C.; Sitbon, K.; Madec, Y.; Denoeud-Ndam, L.; Wolff, M.; Fontanet, A.; Bretagne, S.; Dromer, F. Worrisome trends in incidence and mortality of candidemia in intensive care units (Paris area, 2002–2010). *Intensiv. Care Med.* **2014**, *40*, 1303–1312. [CrossRef]
10. Kullberg, B.J.; Arendrup, M.C. Invasive Candidiasis. *New Engl. J. Med.* **2015**, *373*, 1445–1456. [CrossRef]
11. Marra, A.R.; Camargo, L.F.A.; Pignatari, A.C.C.; Sukiennik, T.; Behar, P.R.P.; Medeiros, E.A.S.; Ribeiro, J.; Girão, E.; Correa, L.; Guerra, C.; et al. Nosocomial Bloodstream Infections in Brazilian Hospitals: Analysis of 2,563 Cases from a Prospective Nationwide Surveillance Study. *J. Clin. Microbiol.* **2011**, *49*, 1866–1871. [CrossRef] [PubMed]
12. Lamoth, F.; Lockhart, S.R.; Berkow, E.L.; Calandra, T. Changes in the epidemiological landscape of invasive candidiasis. *J. Antimicrob. Chemother.* **2018**, *73*, i4–i13. [CrossRef] [PubMed]
13. A Pfaller, M.; Diekema, D.J.; Turnidge, J.D.; Castanheira, M.; Jones, R.N. Twenty Years of the SENTRY Antifungal Surveillance Program: Results for Candida Species from 1997–2016. *Open Forum Infect. Dis.* **2019**, *6*, S79–S94. [CrossRef]
14. Kelley, R.; Healey, D.S.P. Fungal Resistance to Echinocandins and the MDR Phenomenon in Candida glabrata. *J. Fungi* **2018**, *4*, 105. [CrossRef]

15. A Chow, N.; Gade, L.; Tsay, S.V.; Forsberg, K.; A Greenko, J.; Southwick, K.L.; Barrett, P.M.; Kerins, J.L.; Lockhart, S.R.; Chiller, T.M.; et al. Multiple introductions and subsequent transmission of multidrug-resistant Candida auris in the USA: A molecular epidemiological survey. *Lancet Infect. Dis.* **2018**, *18*, 1377–1384. [CrossRef]
16. Eyre, D.W.; Sheppard, A.E.; Madder, H.; Moir, I.; Moroney, R.; Quan, T.P.; Griffiths, D.; George, S.; Butcher, L.; Morgan, M.; et al. A Candida auris Outbreak and Its Control in an Intensive Care Setting. *New Engl. J. Med.* **2018**, *379*, 1322–1331. [CrossRef]
17. Arastehfar, A.; Daneshnia, F.; Hilmioğlu-Polat, S.; Fang, W.; Yaşar, M.; Polat, F.; Metin, D.Y.; Rigole, P.; Coenye, T.; Ilkit, M.; et al. First report of candidemia clonal outbreak caused by emerging fluconazole-resistant Candida parapsilosis isolates harboring Y132F and/or Y132F+K143R in Turkey. *Antimicrob. Agents Chemother.* **2020**. [CrossRef]
18. Available online: https://www.who.int/docs/default-source/coronaviruse/situation-reports/20200718-covid-19-sitrep-180.pdf?sfvrsn=39b31718_2 (accessed on 18 July 2020).
19. Arastehfar, A.; Carvalho, A.; Van De Veerdonk, F.L.; Jenks, J.D.; Köhler, P.; Krause, R.; Cornely, O.A.; Perlin, D.S.; Lass-Flörl, C.; Hoenigl, M. COVID-19 Associated Pulmonary Aspergillosis (CAPA)—From Immunology to Treatment. *J. Fungi* **2020**, *6*, 91. [CrossRef]
20. Chen, N.; Zhou, M.; Dong, X.; Qu, J.; Gong, F.; Han, Y.; Qiu, Y.; Wang, J.; Liu, Y.; Wei, Y.; et al. Epidemiological and clinical characteristics of 99 cases of 2019 novel coronavirus pneumonia in Wuhan, China: A descriptive study. *Lancet* **2020**, *395*, 507–513. [CrossRef]
21. Ventoulis, I.; Sarmourli, T.; Amoiridou, P.; Mantzana, P.; Exindari, M.; Gioula, G.; Vyzantiadis, T.-A. Bloodstream Infection by Saccharomyces cerevisiae in Two COVID-19 Patients after Receiving Supplementation of Saccharomyces in the ICU. *J. Fungi* **2020**, *6*, 98. [CrossRef]
22. Salehi, M.; Ahmadikia, K.; Mahmoudi, S.; Kalantari, S.; Siahkali, S.J.; Izadi, A.; Kord, M.; Manshadi, S.A.D.; Seifi, A.; Ghiasvand, F.; et al. Oropharyngeal candidiasis in hospitalized COVID-19 Patients from Iran: Species identification and antifungal susceptibility pattern. *Mycoses* **2020**. [CrossRef] [PubMed]
23. White, P.L.; Dhillon, R.; Cordey, A.; Hughes, H.; Faggian, F.; Soni, S.; Pandey, M.; Whitaker, H.; May, A.; Morgan, M.; et al. A national strategy to diagnose COVID-19 associated invasive fungal disease in the ICU. *Clin. Infect. Dis.* **2020**. [CrossRef] [PubMed]
24. Posteraro, B.; Torelli, R.; Vella, A.; Leone, P.M.; De Angelis, G.; De Carolis, E.; Ventura, G.; Sanguinetti, M.; Fantoni, M. Pan-Echinocandin-Resistant Candida glabrata Bloodstream Infection Complicating COVID-19: A Fatal Case Report. *J. Fungi* **2020**, *6*, 163. [CrossRef] [PubMed]
25. Al-Hatmi, A.M.; Mohsin, J.; Al-Huraizi, A.; Khamis, F. COVID-19 associated invasive candidiasis. *J. Infect.* **2020**. [CrossRef]
26. Antinori, S.; Bonazzetti, C.; Gubertini, G.; Capetti, A.; Pagani, C.; Morena, V.; Rimoldi, S.; Galimberti, L.; Sarzi-Puttini, P.; Ridolfo, A.L. Tocilizumab for cytokine storm syndrome in COVID-19 pneumonia: An increased risk for candidemia? *Autoimmun. Rev.* **2020**, *19*, 102564. [CrossRef]
27. Chowdhary, A.; Tarai, B.; Singh, A.; Sharma, A. Multidrug-Resistant Candida auris Infections in Critically Ill Coronavirus Disease Patients, India, April–July 2020. *Emerg. Infect. Dis.* **2020**, *26*. [CrossRef]
28. Kuba, K.; Imai, Y.; Rao, S.; Gao, H.; Guo, F.; Guan, B.; Huan, Y.; Yang, P.; Zhang, Y.; Deng, W.; et al. A crucial role of angiotensin converting enzyme 2 (ACE2) in SARS coronavirus-induced lung injury. *Nat. Med.* **2020**, *11*, 875–879. [CrossRef]
29. Glowacka, I.; Bertram, S.; Müller, M.A.; Allen, P.; Soilleux, E.; Pfefferle, S.; Steffen, I.; Tsegaye, T.S.; He, Y.; Gnirss, K.; et al. Evidence that TMPRSS2 Activates the Severe Acute Respiratory Syndrome Coronavirus Spike Protein for Membrane Fusion and Reduces Viral Control by the Humoral Immune Response. *J. Virol.* **2011**, *85*, 4122–4134. [CrossRef]
30. Imai, Y.; Kuba, K.; Rao, S.; Huan, Y.; Guo, F.; Guan, B.; Yang, P.; Sarao, R.; Wada, T.; Leong-Poi, H.; et al. Angiotensin-converting enzyme 2 protects from severe acute lung failure. *Nat. Cell Biol.* **2005**, *436*, 112–116. [CrossRef]
31. Marshall, R.P.; Webb, S.; Bellingan, G.J.; Montgomery, H.; Chaudhari, B.; McAnulty, R.J.; Humphries, S.E.; Hill, M.R.; Laurent, G.J. Angiotensin Converting Enzyme Insertion/Deletion Polymorphism Is Associated with Susceptibility and Outcome in Acute Respiratory Distress Syndrome. *Am. J. Respir. Crit. Care Med.* **2002**, *166*, 646–650. [CrossRef]

32. Mancia, G.; Rea, F.; Ludergnani, M.; Apolone, G.; Corrao, G. Renin–Angiotensin–Aldosterone System Blockers and the Risk of Covid-19. *N. Engl. J. Med.* **2020**, *382*, 2431–2440. [CrossRef] [PubMed]
33. Van De Veerdonk, F.L.; Netea, M.G.; Van Deuren, M.; Van Der Meer, J.W.; De Mast, Q.; Brüggemann, R.J.; Van Der Hoeven, H. Kallikrein-kinin blockade in patients with COVID-19 to prevent acute respiratory distress syndrome. *eLife* **2020**, *9*. [CrossRef] [PubMed]
34. Liao, M.; Liu, Y.; Yuan, J.; Wen, Y.; Xu, G.; Zhao, J.; Cheng, L.; Li, J.; Wang, X.; Wang, F.; et al. Single-cell landscape of bronchoalveolar immune cells in patients with COVID-19. *Nat. Med.* **2020**, *26*, 842–844. [CrossRef] [PubMed]
35. Zheng, M.; Gao, Y.; Wang, G.; Song, G.; Liu, S.; Sun, D.; Xu, Y.; Tian, Z. Functional exhaustion of antiviral lymphocytes in COVID-19 patients. *Cell. Mol. Immunol.* **2020**, *17*, 533–535. [CrossRef]
36. Giamarellos-Bourboulis, E.J.; Netea, M.G.; Rovina, N.; Akinosoglou, K.; Antoniadou, A.; Antonakos, N.; Damoraki, G.; Gkavogianni, T.; Adami, M.-E.; Katsaounou, P.; et al. Complex Immune Dysregulation in COVID-19 Patients with Severe Respiratory Failure. *Cell Host Microbe* **2020**, *27*, 992–1000. [CrossRef]
37. Garcia-Vidal, C.; Sanjuan, G.; Moreno-García, E.; Puerta-Alcalde, P.; Garcia-Pouton, N.; Chumbita, M.; Fernandez-Pittol, M.; Pitart, C.; Inciarte, A.; Bodro, M.; et al. Incidence of co-infections and superinfections in hospitalised patients with COVID-19: A retrospective cohort study. *Clin. Microbiol. Infect.* **2020**. [CrossRef]
38. Hoenigl, M.; Lin, J.; Finkelman, M.; Zhang, Y.; Karris, M.Y.; Letendre, S.; Ellis, R.J.; Burke, L.; Richard, B.; Gaufin, T.; et al. Glucan rich nutrition does not increase gut translocation of Beta glucan. *Mycoses* **2020**. [CrossRef]
39. Leelahavanichkul, A.; Worasilchai, N.; Wannalerdsakun, S.; Jutivorakool, K.; Somparn, P.; Issara-Amphorn, J.; Tachaboon, S.; Srisawat, N.; Finkelman, M.; Chindamporn, A. Gastrointestinal Leakage Detected by Serum (1→3)-β-D-Glucan in Mouse Models and a Pilot Study in Patients with Sepsis. *Shock* **2016**, *46*, 506–518. [CrossRef]
40. Auld, S.C.; Caridi-Scheible, M.; Blum, J.M.; Robichaux, C.J.; Kraft, C.S.; Jacob, J.T.; Jabaley, C.S.; Carpenter, D.; Kaplow, R.; Hernandez, A.C.; et al. ICU and ventilator mortality among critically ill adults with COVID-19. *MedRxiv* **2020**. [CrossRef]
41. Auld, S.C.; Caridi-Scheible, M.; Blum, J.M.; Robichaux, C.; Kraft, C.; Jacob, J.T.; Jabaley, C.S.; Carpenter, D.; Kaplow, R.; Hernandez-Romieu, A.C.; et al. ICU and Ventilator Mortality Among Critically Ill Adults With Coronavirus Disease 2019. *Crit. Care Med.* **2020**, *48*, e799–e804. [CrossRef]
42. Arastehfar, A.; Daneshnia, F.; Hafez, A.; Khodavaisy, S.; Najafzadeh, M.-J.; Charsizadeh, A.; Zarrinfar, H.; Salehi, M.; Shahrabadi, Z.Z.; Sasani, E.; et al. Antifungal susceptibility, genotyping, resistance mechanism, and clinical profile of Candida tropicalis blood isolates. *Med. Mycol.* **2019**, *58*, 766–773. [CrossRef] [PubMed]
43. Ko, J.-H.; Jung, D.S.; Lee, J.Y.; Kim, H.A.; Ryu, S.Y.; Jung, S.-I.; Joo, E.-J.; Cheon, S.; Kim, Y.-S.; Kim, S.-W.; et al. Poor prognosis of Candida tropicalis among non-albicans candidemia: A retrospective multicenter cohort study, Korea. *Diagn. Microbiol. Infect. Dis.* **2019**, *95*, 195–200. [CrossRef] [PubMed]
44. Arastehfar, A.; Lass-Flörl, C.; Garcia-Rubio, R.; Daneshnia, F.; Ilkit, M.; Boekhout, T.; Gabaldón, T.; Perlin, D.S. The Quiet and Underappreciated Rise of Drug-Resistant Invasive Fungal Pathogens. *J. Fungi* **2020**, *6*, 138. [CrossRef] [PubMed]
45. Arastehfar, A.; Hilmioğlu-Polat, S.; Daneshnia, F.; Hafez, A.; Salehi, M.; Polat, F.; Yaşar, M.; Arslan, N.; Hoşbul, T.; Ünal, N.; et al. Recent increase in the prevalence of fluconazole-non-susceptible Candida tropicalis blood isolates in Turkey: Clinical implication of azolenon- susceptible and fluconazole tolerant phenotypes and genotyping. *Front. Microbiol.* **2020**, *11*, 2383. [CrossRef]
46. Berman, J.; Krysan, D.J. Drug resistance and tolerance in fungi. *Nat. Rev. Genet.* **2020**, *18*, 319–331. [CrossRef]
47. Schelenz, S. Management of candidiasis in the intensive care unit. *J. Antimicrob. Chemother.* **2008**, *61*, i31–i34. [CrossRef]
48. Pappas, P.G.; Lionakis, M.S.; Arendrup, M.C.; Ostrosky-Zeichner, L.; Kullberg, B.J. Invasive candidiasis. *Nat. Rev. Dis. Prim.* **2018**, *4*, 18026. [CrossRef]
49. Pittiruti, M.; Pinelli, F. Recommendations for the use of vascular access in the COVID-19 patients: An Italian perspective. *Crit. Care* **2020**, *24*, 1–3. [CrossRef]
50. Chowdhary, A.; Sharma, A. The lurking scourge of multidrug resistant Candida auris in times of COVID-19 pandemic. *J. Glob. Antimicrob. Resist.* **2020**, *22*, 175–176. [CrossRef]

51. Tóth, R.; Nosek, J.; Mora-Montes, H.M.; Gabaldon, T.; Bliss, J.M.; Nosanchuk, J.D.; Turner, S.A.; Butler, G.; Vágvölgyi, C.; Gácser, A. Candida parapsilosis: From Genes to the Bedside. *Clin. Microbiol. Rev.* **2019**, *32*. [CrossRef]
52. Arastehfar, A.; Daneshnia, F.; Hilmioglu-Polat, S.; Ilkit, M.; Yasar, M.; Polat, F.; Metin, D.Y.; Dokumcu, Ü.Z.; Pan, W.; Hagen, F.; et al. Genetically-related micafungin-resistant C. parapsilosis blood isolates harboring a novel mutation R658G in hotspot1-Fks1p: A new challenge? *J. Antimicrob. Chemother.* **2020**, submitted.
53. Arastehfar, A.; Daneshnia, F.; Najafzadeh, M.J.; Hagen, F.; Mahmoudi, S.; Salehi, M.; Zarrinfar, H.; Namvar, Z.; Zareshahrabadi, Z.; Khodavaisy, S.; et al. Evaluation of Molecular Epidemiology, Clinical Characteristics, Antifungal Susceptibility Profiles, and Molecular Mechanisms of Antifungal Resistance of Iranian Candida parapsilosis Species Complex Blood Isolates. *Front. Cell. Infect. Microbiol.* **2020**, *10*, 206. [CrossRef] [PubMed]
54. Ben-Ami, R.; Olshtain-Pops, K.; Krieger, M.; Oren, I.; Bishara, J.; Dan, M.; Wiener-Well, Y.; Weinberger, M.; Zimhony, O.; Chowers, M.; et al. Antibiotic Exposure as a Risk Factor for Fluconazole-Resistant Candida Bloodstream Infection. *Antimicrob. Agents Chemother.* **2012**, *56*, 2518–2523. [CrossRef] [PubMed]
55. Lin, M.Y.; Carmeli, Y.; Zumsteg, J.; Flores, E.L.; Tolentino, J.; Sreeramoju, P.; Weber, S.G. Prior Antimicrobial Therapy and Risk for Hospital-Acquired Candida glabrata and Candida krusei Fungemia: A Case-Case-Control Study. *Antimicrob. Agents Chemother.* **2005**, *49*, 4555–4560. [CrossRef]
56. Pittet, D.; Monod, M.; Suter, P.M.; Frenk, E.; Auckenthaler, R. Candida colonization and subsequent infections in critically ill surgical patients. *Ann. Surg.* **1994**, *220*, 751–758. [CrossRef]
57. Romo, J.A.; Kumamoto, C.A. On Commensalism of Candida. *J. Fungi* **2020**, *6*, 16. [CrossRef]
58. Bertolini, M.; Ranjan, A.; Thompson, A.; Diaz, P.I.; Sobue, T.; Maas, K.; Dongari-Bagtzoglou, A. Candida albicans induces mucosal bacterial dysbiosis that promotes invasive infection. *PLoS Pathog.* **2019**, *15*, e1007717. [CrossRef]
59. Mason, K.L.; Downward, J.R.E.; Mason, K.D.; Falkowski, N.R.; Eaton, K.A.; Kao, J.Y.; Young, V.B.; Huffnagle, G.B. Candida albicans and Bacterial Microbiota Interactions in the Cecum during Recolonization following Broad-Spectrum Antibiotic Therapy. *Infect. Immun.* **2013**, *80*, 3371–3380. [CrossRef]
60. Issara-Amphorn, J.; Surawut, S.; Worasilchai, N.; Thim-Uam, A.; Finkelman, M.; Chindamporn, A.; Palaga, T.; Hirankarn, N.; Pisitkun, P.; Leelahavanichkul, A. The Synergy of Endotoxin and (1→3)-β-D-Glucan, from Gut Translocation, Worsens Sepsis Severity in a Lupus Model of Fc Gamma Receptor IIb-Deficient Mice. *J. Innat. Immun.* **2018**, *10*, 189–201. [CrossRef]
61. Hoenigl, M. Fungal Translocation: A driving force behind the Occurrence of non-AIDS Events? *Clin. Infect. Dis.* **2019**, *70*, 242–244. [CrossRef]
62. Leelahavanichkul, A.; Panpetch, W.; Worasilchai, N.; Somparn, P.; Chancharoenthana, W.; Nilgate, S.; Finkelman, M.; Chindamporn, A.; Tumwasorn, S. Evaluation of gastrointestinal leakage using serum (1–>3)-beta-D-glucan in a Clostridium difficile murine model. *FEMS Microbiol. Lett.* **2016**, *363*, fnw204. [CrossRef] [PubMed]
63. Cavayas, Y.A.; Yusuff, H.; Porter, R. Fungal infections in adult patients on extracorporeal life support. *Crit. Care* **2018**, *22*, 98. [CrossRef] [PubMed]
64. Clancy, C.J.; Nguyen, M.H. Diagnosing Invasive Candidiasis. *J. Clin. Microbiol.* **2018**, *56*, e01909-17. [CrossRef] [PubMed]
65. Arastehfar, A.; Wickes, B.L.; Ilkit, M.; Pincus, D.H.; Daneshnia, F.; Pan, W.; Fang, W.; Boekhout, T. Identification of Mycoses in Developing Countries. *J. Fungi* **2019**, *5*, 90. [CrossRef]
66. Onishi, A.; Sugiyama, D.; Kogata, Y.; Saegusa, J.; Sugimoto, T.; Kawano, S.; Morinobu, A.; Nishimura, K.; Kumagai, S. Diagnostic accuracy of serum 1,3-β-D-glucan for pneumocystis jiroveci pneumonia, invasive candidiasis, and invasive aspergillosis: Systematic review and meta-analysis. *J. Clin. Microbiol.* **2012**, *50*, 7–15. [CrossRef]
67. Karageorgopoulos, D.E.; Vouloumanou, E.K.; Ntziora, F.; Michalopoulos, A.; I Rafailidis, P.; Falagas, M. β-D-glucan assay for the diagnosis of invasive fungal infections: A meta-analysis. *Clin. Infect. Dis.* **2011**, *52*, 750–770. [CrossRef]
68. Giacobbe, D.R.; Mikulska, M.; Tumbarello, M.; Furfaro, E.; Spadaro, M.; Losito, A.R.; Mesini, A.; De Pascale, G.; Marchese, A.; Bruzzone, M.; et al. Combined use of serum (1,3)-β-D-glucan and procalcitonin for the early differential diagnosis between candidaemia and bacteraemia in intensive care units. *Crit. Care* **2017**, *21*, 176. [CrossRef]

69. Yang, A.-M.; Inamine, T.; Hochrath, K.; Chen, P.; Wang, L.; Llorente, C.; Bluemel, S.; Hartmann, P.; Xu, J.; Koyama, Y.; et al. Intestinal fungi contribute to development of alcoholic liver disease. *J. Clin. Investig.* **2017**, *127*, 2829–2841. [CrossRef]
70. Prattes, J.; Hoenigl, M.; Rabensteiner, J.; Raggam, R.B.; Prueller, F.; Zollner-Schwetz, I.; Valentin, T.; Hönigl, K.; Fruhwald, S.; Krause, R. Serum 1,3-beta-d-glucan for antifungal treatment stratification at the intensive care unit and the influence of surgery. *Mycoses* **2014**, *57*, 679–686. [CrossRef]
71. Posteraro, B.; Tumbarello, M.; De Pascale, G.; Liberto, E.; Vallecoccia, M.S.; De Carolis, E.; Di Gravio, V.; Trecarichi, E.M.; Sanguinetti, M.; Antonelli, M. (1,3)-β-d-Glucan-based antifungal treatment in critically ill adults at high risk of candidaemia: An observational study. *J. Antimicrob. Chemother.* **2016**, *71*, 2262–2269. [CrossRef]
72. Mikulska, M.; Calandra, T.; Sanguinetti, M.; Poulain, D.; Viscoli, C. The use of mannan antigen and anti-mannan antibodies in the diagnosis of invasive candidiasis: Recommendations from the Third European Conference on Infections in Leukemia. *Crit. Care* **2010**, *14*, R222. [CrossRef] [PubMed]
73. Avni, T.; Leibovici, L.; Paul, M. PCR diagnosis of invasive candidiasis: Systematic review and meta-analysis. *J. Clin. Microbiol.* **2011**, *49*, 665–670. [CrossRef] [PubMed]
74. Zurl, C.J.; Prattes, J.; Zollner-Schwetz, I.; Valentin, T.; Rabensteiner, J.; Wunsch, S.; Hoenigl, M.; Krause, R. T2Candida magnetic resonance in patients with invasive candidiasis: Strengths and limitations. *Med. Mycol.* **2020**, *58*, 632–638. [CrossRef] [PubMed]
75. Clancy, C.J.; Pappas, P.G.; Vazquez, J.; Judson, M.A.; Kontoyiannis, D.P.; Thompson, G.R.; Garey, K.W.; Reboli, A.; Greenberg, R.N.; Apewokin, S.; et al. Detecting Infections Rapidly and Easily for Candidemia Trial, Part 2 (DIRECT2): A Prospective, Multicenter Study of the T2Candida Panel. *Clin. Infect. Dis.* **2018**, *66*, 1678–1686. [CrossRef] [PubMed]
76. Lamoth, F.; Clancy, C.J.; Tissot, F.; Squires, K.; Eggimann, P.; Flückiger, U.; Siegemund, M.; Orasch, C.; Zimmerli, S.; Calandra, T.; et al. Performance of the T2Candida Panel for the Diagnosis of Intra-abdominal Candidiasis. *Open Forum Infect. Dis.* **2020**, *7*, ofaa075. [CrossRef] [PubMed]
77. Calandra, T.; Roberts, J.A.; Antonelli, M.; Bassetti, M.; Vincent, J.-L. Diagnosis and management of invasive candidiasis in the ICU: An updated approach to an old enemy. *Crit. Care* **2016**, *20*, 125. [CrossRef] [PubMed]
78. Nguyen, M.H.; Wissel, M.C.; Shields, R.K.; Salomoni, M.A.; Hao, B.; Press, E.G.; Cheng, S.; Mitsani, D.; Vadnerkar, A.; Silveira, F.P.; et al. Performance of Candida real-time polymerase chain reaction, β-D-glucan assay, and blood cultures in the diagnosis of invasive candidiasis. *Clin. Infect. Dis.* **2012**, *54*, 1240–1248. [CrossRef]
79. Koehler, P.; Arendrup, M.C.; Arikan-Akdagli, S.; Bassetti, M.; Bretagne, S.; Klingspor, L.; Lagrou, K.; Meis, J.F.; Rautemaa-Richardson, R.; Schelenz, S.; et al. ECMM CandiReg-A ready to use platform for outbreaks and epidemiological studies. *Mycoses* **2019**, *62*, 920–927. [CrossRef]
80. A Cornely, O.; Bassetti, M.; Calandra, T.; Garbino, J.; Kullberg, B.; Lortholary, O.; Meersseman, W.; Akova, M.; Arendrup, M.; Arikan-Akdagli, S.; et al. ESCMID* guideline for the diagnosis and management of Candida diseases 2012: Non-neutropenic adult patients. *Clin. Microbiol. Infect.* **2012**, *18*, 19–37. [CrossRef]
81. Pappas, P.G.; Kauffman, C.A.; Andes, D.R.; Clancy, C.J.; Marr, K.A.; Ostrosky-Zeichner, L.; Reboli, A.C.; Schuster, M.G.; Vazquez, J.A.; Walsh, T.J.; et al. Clinical Practice Guideline for the Management of Candidiasis: 2016 Update by the Infectious Diseases Society of America. *Clin. Infect. Dis.* **2016**, *62*, e1–e50. [CrossRef]
82. Cornely, O.A.; Hoenigl, M.; Lass-Flörl, C.; Chen SC, A.; Kontoyiannis, D.P.; Morrissey, C.O.; Thompson, G.R., III. Defining breakthrough invasive fungal infection-Position paper of the mycoses study group education and research consortium and the European Confederation of Medical Mycology. *Mycoses* **2019**, *62*, 716–729. [CrossRef] [PubMed]
83. Aruanno, M.; Glampedakis, E.; Lamoth, F. Echinocandins for the Treatment of Invasive Aspergillosis: From Laboratory to Bedside. *Antimicrob. Agents Chemother.* **2019**, *63*, e00399-19. [CrossRef] [PubMed]
84. Zhao, Y.; Prideaux, B.; Nagasaki, Y.; Lee, M.H.; Chen, P.-Y.; Blanc, L.; Ho, H.; Clancy, C.J.; Nguyen, M.H.; Dartois, V.; et al. Unraveling Drug Penetration of Echinocandin Antifungals at the Site of Infection in an Intra-abdominal Abscess Model. *Antimicrob. Agents Chemother.* **2017**, *61*, e01009-17. [CrossRef] [PubMed]

Journal of *Fungi*

MDPI

Case Report

Pan-Echinocandin-Resistant *Candida glabrata* Bloodstream Infection Complicating COVID-19: A Fatal Case Report

Brunella Posteraro [1,2,†], Riccardo Torelli [3,†], Antonietta Vella [3,†], Paolo Maria Leone [2], Giulia De Angelis [1,3], Elena De Carolis [3], Giulio Ventura [3,4], Maurizio Sanguinetti [1,3,*] and Massimo Fantoni [3,4]

1 Dipartimento di Scienze Biotecnologiche di Base, Cliniche Intensivologiche e Perioperatorie, Università Cattolica del Sacro Cuore, 00168 Rome, Italy; brunella.posteraro@unicatt.it (B.P.); giulia.deangelis78@gmail.com (G.D.A.)

2 Dipartimento di Scienze Gastroenterologiche, Endocrino-Metaboliche e Nefro-Urologiche, Fondazione Policlinico Universitario A. Gemelli IRCCS, 00168 Rome, Italy; paolomaria.leone@policlinicogemelli.it

3 Dipartimento di Scienze di Laboratorio e Infettivologiche, Fondazione Policlinico Universitario A. Gemelli IRCCS, 00168 Rome, Italy; riccardo.torelli@policlinicogemelli.it (R.T.); antonietta.vella@policlinicogemelli.it (A.V.); elena.decarolis@policlinicogemelli.it (E.D.C.); giulio.ventura@unicatt.it (G.V.); massimo.fantoni@unicatt.it (M.F.)

4 Dipartimento di Sicurezza e Bioetica, Università Cattolica del Sacro Cuore, 00168 Rome, Italy

* Correspondence: maurizio.sanguinetti@unicatt.it; Tel.: +39-6-305-4411

† These authors contributed equally to this work.

Received: 6 August 2020; Accepted: 4 September 2020; Published: 6 September 2020

Abstract: Coinfections with bacteria or fungi may be a frequent complication of COVID-19, but coinfections with *Candida* species in COVID-19 patients remain rare. We report the 53-day clinical course of a complicated type-2 diabetes patient diagnosed with COVID-19, who developed bloodstream infections initially due to methicillin-resistant *Staphylococcus aureus*, secondly due to multidrug-resistant Gram-negative bacteria, and lastly due to a possibly fatal *Candida glabrata*. The development of *FKS*-associated pan-echinocandin resistance in the *C. glabrata* isolated from the patient after 13 days of caspofungin treatment aggravated the situation. The patient died of septic shock shortly before the prospect of receiving potentially effective antifungal therapy. This case emphasizes the importance of early diagnosis and monitoring for antimicrobial drug-resistant coinfections to reduce their unfavorable outcomes in COVID-19 patients.

Keywords: SARS-CoV-2; coinfection; diabetes; bloodstream infection; *Candida glabrata*; echinocandin resistance; *FKS* mutation

1. Introduction

Since the beginning of the respiratory tract infection epidemic in China [1] caused by the 2019 severe acute respiratory syndrome coronavirus 2 (SARS-CoV-2), known as coronavirus disease 2019 (COVID-19), a substantial number of COVID-19 associated deaths have been reported worldwide [2]. While sepsis may be a fatal complication of COVID-19 [3], coinfection (also named superinfection) with bacteria or fungi may occur, albeit confined to the respiratory tract [4,5]. In two independent studies from Chinese hospitals, 27 (96.4%) of 28 [6] and 11 (16%) of 68 [7] COVID-19 patients who died had secondary infections. This is consistent with failed homeostasis between innate and adaptive responses [8] or a pronounced immune suppression [9], which is partly dependent on the loss of lymphocytes, following SARS-CoV-2 infection [10]. Diabetes is the most common comorbidity in

COVID-19, with its late complications (e.g., ischemic heart disease) contributing to further increases in COVID-19 severity [11]. Additionally, diabetes increases not only the risk of infections [11] but also that of infection-related deaths [12]. In this context, diabetes seems to alter the intestinal barrier function, allowing gut microbiota members (e.g., *Enterobacterales* or *Candida* species) to reach the bloodstream and then to spread systemically [13].

Unlike invasive pulmonary aspergillosis, which has emerged as a secondary disease in COVID-19 patients with acute respiratory distress syndrome (ARDS) [14], invasive fungal diseases such as candidiasis and/or candidemia seem to be underestimated in the context of COVID-19. This is surprising, particularly when thinking of *Candida glabrata* [15], a common fungal commensal living on mucosal surfaces, which is the second leading cause of bloodstream infection (candidemia) in some countries, including the USA, Asia and European countries [16,17]. Among *Candida* species displaying multidrug resistance (e.g., co-resistance to azoles and echinocandins), *C. glabrata* is also known for its high tolerance to antifungal drugs [15]. Additionally, as this species has a tropism that causes candidemia among the elderly, COVID-19 patients suffering from ARDS (who are mostly elderly) could be prone to developing candidemia due to *C. glabrata*. This will be of particular concern in the case of COVID-19 patients with candidemia caused by echinocandin-resistant *C. glabrata*, because this species is intrinsically less azole susceptible, and consequently, the use of polyene antifungal drugs (i.e., amphotericin B) due to renal toxicity is largely limited among the elderly. It is noteworthy that COVID-19 itself is associated with kidney injury, which may further hamper the utility of amphotericin B in this context.

We describe the case of a COVID-19 patient with complicated type-2 diabetes who developed a bloodstream infection due to a *Candida glabrata* isolate that acquired pan-echinocandin resistance after 13 days of caspofungin treatment. The patient died of septic shock in the intensive care unit (ICU), shortly before the prospect of receiving potentially effective antifungal therapy.

2. Case Report and Results

A 79-year-old male presented to the emergency department in April 2020 with cough and dyspnea, following a suspected COVID-19 diagnosis because of his previous contact with a SARS-CoV-2 positive patient in a rehabilitation facility. Two days prior to admission (defined as day 1), he had been suffering from fever (38.0 °C). His 6-year medical history was significant for poorly controlled type-2 diabetes, ischemic heart disease and a stadium IV (necrosis and/or gangrene of the limb) peripheral artery disease treated with lower extremity revascularization, which culminated in left leg amputation in 2019. On physical examination, the amputated leg stump displayed necrotic and ulcerative lesions, whereas the patient was afebrile and negative for abnormal lung sounds and had a 98% blood oxygenation. His leucocytes ($\times 10^9$/L) were normal (4.7; normal range 4.0–10.0), whereas his serum creatinine (mg/dL) (1.3; normal range 0.7–1.2), C-reactive protein (CRP, mg/L) (37.8; normal range 0.0–5.0) and interleukin 6 (IL6, ng/L) (13.6; normal range 0.0–4.4) were altered. The patient's chest X-ray and computed tomography findings were consistent with pneumonia, and positive SARS-CoV-2 RNA detection results (C_T 30.3; E gene [18]) on nasal/pharyngeal swabs obtained in the emergency department allowed confirmation of the COVID-19 diagnosis [19]. Subsequent nasal/pharyngeal swabs taken from the patient at different times from admission tested positive for SARS-CoV-2 RNA.

The patient was transferred to the COVID-19 care unit, where he was started on antiviral therapy (which was continued for the next five days) with darunavir/ritonavir (800/100 mg q24h) combined with hydroxychloroquine (200 mg q12h), which was our national policy at that time. On days 4 and 5, the patient's clinical conditions worsened, and his serum creatinine, CRP and leukocytes increased to 3.5 mg/dL, 155.4 mg/L and 6.9×10^9/L, respectively. The patient developed fever (38.2 °C), a productive cough, and his blood oxygenation decreased to 92%, demanding oxygen administration through a Venturi mask (fraction of inspired oxygen, 24%). Due to highly suspected bacterial superinfection, he received empirical treatment with piperacillin/tazobactam (2.25 g q6h).

On day 8, the patient was still febrile (38.5 °C), his serum creatinine (3.9 mg/dL), CRP (177.2 mg/L) and leukocytes (9.4×10^9/L) rose further, and his blood cultures from day 5 grew a methicillin-resistant *Staphylococcus aureus* organism. Consequently, piperacillin/tazobactam was discontinued and teicoplanin (200 mg q24h) was started. He improved, and subsequent blood cultures, a transthoracic echocardiogram and ultrasound studies to evaluate deep vein thrombosis were all negative. On day 25, teicoplanin was discontinued. The next day, both orthopedic and vascular surgeons who evaluated the patient decided on a new, more proximal amputation of his left leg. On day 27, the patient became febrile (38.5 °C). His leukocytes increased to 10.8×10^9/L and infection indexes, including procalcitonin (PCT; normal range, 0.0–0.5 ng/mL), were elevated (CRP, 275 mg/L; PCT, 1.65 ng/mL). While his kidney injury seemed to recover (serum creatinine, 1.5 mg/dL), the patient became stably anemic (hemoglobin, g/dL; 7.4; normal range 13.0–17.0), requiring regular blood transfusions (until two days before death). On day 28, blood cultures from day 27 grew *Morganella morganii* (found to be resistant to cephalosporins and piperacillin/tazobactam but susceptible to carbapenems), which prompted initiation of antibiotic therapy with ertapenem (1 g q24h). Concomitantly, cultures from a progressively enlarging ulcer on the patient's leg stump revealed growth of *Proteus mirabilis*, *Klebsiella pneumoniae* and *Escherichia coli* (all found to be susceptible to carbapenems).

On day 35, the patient again became febrile (38.2 °C) but CRP decreased (177.2 mg/L) and leukocytes remained unchanged (9.3×10^9/L). Blood cultures yielded a yeast organism, later identified as *C. glabrata* using a previously described matrix-assisted laser desorption/ionization time-of-flight (MALDI-TOF) mass spectrometry-based method [20]. The isolate (defined as isolate 1) was susceptible to anidulafungin, micafungin and caspofungin, with MICs of 0.03, 0.03 and 0.06 μg/mL (SensititreYeastOne® method; Thermo Fisher Scientific, Cleveland, OH, USA), according to the Clinical and Laboratory Standards (CLSI) clinical breakpoints [21]. On day 37, the patient started to take caspofungin (70 mg loading dose, day 1; 50 mg q24h, subsequent days). Blood cultures from day 39 were negative. After 13 days of antifungal therapy, the patient became febrile again (38.3 °C), and his blood parameters (creatinine, 2.71 mg/dL; leukocytes, 12.48×10^9/L) and infection indexes (CRP, 278.4 mg/L; PCT, 20.58 ng/mL) were abnormal. On day 49, blood cultures were positive for *Acinetobacter baumannii* (found to be only susceptible to colistin) and again for *C. glabrata*. While ertapenem was discontinued and colistin (2.25 mUI q12h) was started, the patient continued to receive caspofungin. Shortly after (day 51), antifungal susceptibility testing was repeated on two morphologically different *C. glabrata* isolates that grew from blood cultures. One of the isolates (defined as isolate 2) revealed increased MICs of anidulafungin, micafungin and caspofungin, indicating resistance to all echinocandins (as discussed below).

On day 52, the patient underwent surgery for the previously planned left leg re-amputation. Unfortunately, on the same day of surgery and before the patient could eventually benefit from antifungal therapy change (i.e., amphotericin B instead of caspofungin) based on available antifungal susceptibility results, his clinical conditions worsened. The patient was immediately transferred to the ICU due to refractory septic shock, as identified by the receipt of vasopressor therapy and the elevated lactate (mEq/L) level (4.2; normal range 0.0–2.0) despite adequate fluid resuscitation. On day 53, the patient died.

Table 1 summarizes the results of both antifungal susceptibility testing and *FKS2* gene sequencing for *C. glabrata* isolates 1 and 2. Only for echinocandin antifungal agents, MIC values obtained with the SensititreYeastOne® method were confirmed by the CLSI M27-A3 reference method [21]. As noted, except for all three echinocandins, the antifungal susceptibility profile of isolate 2 did not change compared to that of isolate 1. According to the echinocandin-resistant breakpoint values established by the CLSI [18], isolate 2 showed resistance to anidulafungin (MIC, 2 mg/L), caspofungin (MIC, 8 mg/L) and micafungin (MIC, 8 mg/L). Conversely, isolate 1 had echinocandin MICs (anidulafungin and micafungin, 0.03 mg/L; caspofungin, 0.06 mg/L) below the CLSI echinocandin-resistant breakpoint values [22]. Interestingly, both the isolates showed an intermediate susceptibility to fluconazole (MIC, 8 mg/L) and, according to the epidemiological cutoff values established by the CLSI [23], a wild-type susceptibility to amphotericin B, and the other azole (itraconazole, posaconazole and voriconazole) antifungal agents tested. A sequence analysis of the *FKS1*/*FKS2* genes [24] allowed us to identify T1976A (hot spot 1) and A3997T (hot spot 2) mutations in the *FKS2* gene, which resulted in an F659Y or I1333F amino acid change, respectively, with the former being already known [16,25,26] and the latter probably responsible for the observed echinocandin resistance. Furthermore, the MALDI-TOF MS-based analysis of profiles from *C. glabrata* isolates 1 and 2 allowed for comparing them with each other and with profiles from a clinical collection of *C. glabrata* isolates, which had been cultured from sterile or mucosal site samples (UCSC1–12, UCSC17–21). In particular, using the Bruker Daltonics BioTyper 3.0 software, raw spectra from the isolates were matched (with default parameter settings) against the main spectra from an in-house database [20]. Then, the integrated statistical tool Matlab 7.1 of the Biotyper 3.0 software allowed for generating a dendrogram (representation of hierarchical cluster analysis) of spectra to obtain graphical distance values between the isolates. As shown in Figure 1, the dendrogram resulting from the MALDI-TOF MS cluster analysis strongly suggested identity for *C. glabrata* isolates 1 and 2. It is likely that next-generation sequencing analysis could have provided greater discrimination/evidence of similarity among the isolates studied. However, a multilocus sequence-typing scheme (https://pubmlst.org/cglabrata/) showed that isolate 1 was the parental isolate from which originated isolate 2. Indeed, both the isolates shared the sequence type 22 for the analyzed loci *FKS*, *LEU2*, *NMT1*, *TRP1*, *UGP1* and *URA3* (7-5-6-12-1-8).

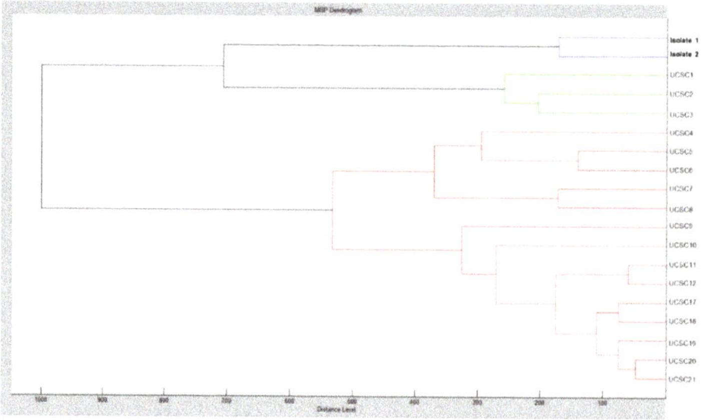

Figure 1. Cluster analysis of matrix-assisted laser desorption/ionization time-of-flight (MALDI-TOF) mass spectra obtained for 19 *C. glabrata* isolates, including the patients' isolates 1 and 2. Shown is a dendrogram in which the distance between isolates is indicated as relative units. Zero means complete similarity and 1000 means complete dissimilarity. An arbitrary distance level of 500 was chosen to assess clustering among isolates.

Table 1. Antifungal susceptibility testing and *FKS2* gene sequencing results of two sequential candidemia isolates.

Species	Isolate	MIC (mg/L) for Polyene Antifungal Class	MIC (mg/L) for Echinocandin Antifungal Class			MIC (mg/L) for Azole Antifungal Class				*FKS2* Gene Hot Spots 1 and 2	
		AMB	AFG	CAS	MFG	FLZ	ITC	POS	VRC	Nucleotide Change	Amino acid Change
C. glabrata	Isolate 1	0.5	0.03	0.06	0.03	8	0.5	1	0.25	Wild type	Wild type
C. glabrata	Isolate 2	0.5	2	8	8	8	0.5	1	0.25	T1976A A3997T C4002T	F659Y I1333F A1334A (wild type)

Abbreviations: MIC, minimum inhibitory concentration; AMB, amphotericin B; AFG, anidulafungin; CAS, caspofungin; MFG, micafungin; FLZ, fluconazole; ITC, itraconazole; POS, posaconazole; VRC, voriconazole. Antifungal-resistant breakpoint values established by the CLSI for *C. glabrata* are ≥0.5 mg/L for anidulafungin and caspofungin, ≥0.25 mg/L for micafungin, and ≥64 mg/L for fluconazole. Because no resistance breakpoints were available for other listed antifungal agents, we used epidemiological cutoff values (ECVs) established by the CLSI for *C. glabrata*, according to which the non-wild-type MIC values (>ECVs) of amphotericin B, itraconazole, posaconazole and voriconazole are >2 mg/L, >4 mg/L, >1 mg/L and >0.25 mg/L, respectively.

3. Discussion

This case illustrates the 53-day clinical course of a COVID-19 patient with persistent SARS-CoV-2 infection (repeated nasal/pharyngeal swabs tested positive for SARS-CoV-2 RNA) who needed protracted hospitalization, probably attributed to his major comorbidity (diabetes with its vascular complications). The patient met the clinical (fever, cough and dyspnea), laboratory (high CRP) and imaging (unilateral pneumonia) features recently recognized as COVID-19 hallmarks [10]. Yet, this case emphasizes the current uncertainty about the clinical disease evolution, partly linked to the presence of risk factors for either admission to the ICU or a fatal outcome of hospitalized patients [10]. In our patient, a succession of bloodstream infections, initially due to methicillin-resistant *S. aureus*, secondly due to multidrug-resistant Gram-negative bacteria, and lastly due to a possibly fatal echinocandin-resistant *C. glabrata*, outlined the COVID-19 associated clinical course (Figure 2).

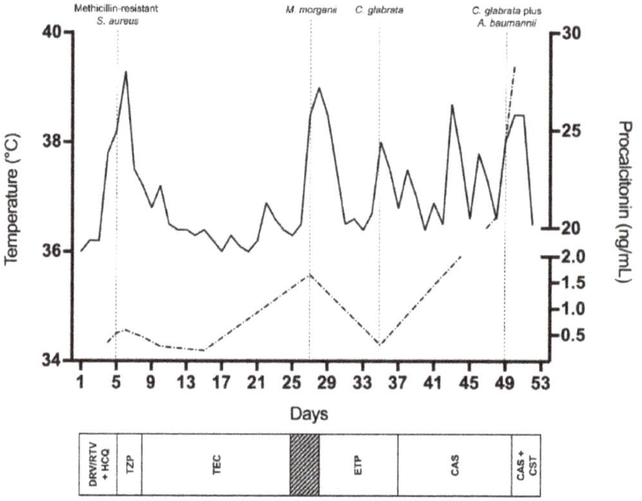

Figure 2. Timeline of major microbiological events during the patient's clinical course and relative antimicrobial treatments. Fever (solid line) or procalcitonin (dashed line) patterns are shown. DRV/RTV, darunavir/ritonavir; HCQ, hydroxychloroquine; TZP; piperacillin/tazobactam; TEC, teicoplanin; ETP, ertapenem; CAS, caspofungin; CST, colistin.

At least three relevant causes might have contributed to determining fatal illness in the present case. First, COVID-19, which has significantly been associated with complications and deaths [10]. Second, type-2 diabetes, which remains a major comorbidity for severe COVID-19 [10,27] and increases the risk of mortality, especially in individuals with poorly controlled blood glucose [28]. Third, superinfection, which represents a new albeit scarcely studied condition in COVID-19 [5], particularly for invasive fungal infections [14,29]. The peculiar pathophysiology of either diabetes [11] or COVID-19 [30] may account for the occurrence of bacterial and fungal coinfections in our case, as in other cases [3,31]. The diabetes-induced immune dysregulation may exacerbate the virus-activated hyper-inflammatory "cytokine storm", which in turn leads to complications (e.g., ARDS, shock, multiorgan failure and death) seen in severe COVID-19 phases [10]. However, diabetes (or other comorbidity) and COVID-19 commonly coexist during patients' hospital stay as risk factors for fungal infection [29], although the extensive use of antibiotics and multiple bacteremias (as in this case) significantly predisposes one to development of candidemia. If candidemia was the immediate cause of death in our patient, it remains a matter of debate considering that the death was preceded by a surgical intervention, which may be relevant to the patient's outcome.

In our patient's disease phase upon his admission to the hospital, COVID-19 together with diabetes might have created a milieu that allowed microorganisms (e.g., *C. glabrata*, the last in the temporal sequence), including those resistant to antimicrobial agents, to thrive (likely in the gastrointestinal tract) and, hence, reach the bloodstream [32,33]. Immunosuppression and mucosal barrier disruption are, among others, well-recognized factors for isolation of *C. glabrata* from patient blood cultures [34] and, to some extent, bloodstream isolates are in vitro resistant to echinocandins [16,25,35]. This poses a great challenge for patient management [36] because echinocandins represent the first line of treatment in cases of invasive *C. glabrata* infections, including candidemia [37], due to the intrinsic low level of *C. glabrata* susceptibility to azoles (which was not the case of our patient's isolates) [22].

Ultimately, the appearance of echinocandin resistance in our patient's *C. glabrata* isolate aggravated the feared adverse prognosis of candidemia [38]. We provided the evidence of an in vivo development of *FKS*-associated echinocandin resistance during the patient's treatment with caspofungin, consistent with previous case reports [26,39,40]. In two of them, echinocandin-resistant isolates were recovered from blood cultures of patients who had recurrent or persistent *C. glabrata* infections, thus implying micafungin treatments for 86 days in one case [26] and 30 days in the other case [39]. In another one [40], echinocandin resistance emerged within 8 days of the patient's treatment with micafungin, and surprisingly, the patient had no previous or prolonged echinocandin exposure [41], but only uncontrolled diabetes, as a potential risk factor for microbiological failure. The abdominal cavity and mucosal surfaces are reservoirs for *Candida* species and a potential source for antifungal resistance due to uneven drug penetration [42,43]. Considering *C. glabrata*'s high propensity for acquiring in vitro resistance following echinocandin exposure [44], it is possible that an underlying gastrointestinal disorder or dysbiosis acted as selectors of *FKS* mutant *C. glabrata* subpopulations in our, as in other [40], case patients. Notably, a study assessing the emergence of in vitro resistance for the three echinocandins showed that 82 of 247 *C. glabrata* breakthrough isolates (i.e., bloodstream isolates exposed to each echinocandin agent) harbored *FKS* hot spot mutations, of which 6 were in *FKS1* and 76 in *FKS2* [45]. Of the three echinocandins, caspofungin seemed to be the most sensitive indicator of *FKS* mutations, whereas only four breakthrough isolates did not develop an *FKS* hot spot mutation despite showing greater than four-fold increases in echinocandin MICs relative to the parental isolates [45]. Of note, the rates of spontaneous *FKS* mutations observed with caspofungin were higher than with anidulafungin or micafungin [45]. Therefore, in our case, the use of caspofungin as a strong inducer of *FKS* mutations may have resulted in the rapid development of echinocandin resistance and subsequent therapeutic failure.

Although non-*FKS*-mediated echinocandin resistance has been reported [46,47], phenotypic resistance (MICs above CLSI breakpoints) to all three echinocandins is uniquely attributable to the presence of mutations in hot spots of both *FKS1* and its paralog *FKS2* [48], which results in attenuated echinocandin activity [49]. As recommended by the current Infectious Diseases Society of America (IDSA) guidelines [37], we performed echinocandin susceptibility testing on the *C. glabrata* isolates causing candidemia in our patient. Thus, we documented that isolate 2 ("breakthrough" isolate), compared to isolate 1 ("parental" isolate), had increased MIC values of anidulafungin, caspofungin and micafungin, and all values were higher than the CLSI resistance breakpoints [22]. As specifically shown for *C. glabrata* and echinocandins [50], the automated blood culture systems currently used to detect bloodstream infections allow for the reliable recovery of isolate populations composed of echinocandin-resistant and echinocandin-susceptible cells. However, in cases with a low proportion of resistant cells, picking up single colonies to perform standard antifungal susceptibility testing may result in missed detections of echinocandin resistance [50]. In our case, taking advantage of morphologically different *C. glabrata* colonies [51] from the patient's blood culture that yielded isolate 2, we were able to detect echinocandin resistance by testing more than one colony. Consistent with recent studies [16,26], we found that isolate 2 harbored the *FKS2* HS1 F659Y. In a two-year antifungal resistance surveillance study [16], 8 (15.7%) of 51 *C. glabrata* isolates with *FKS* HS alterations harbored the *FKS2* HS1 F659S/V/Y [25,52], which was the second found after the *FKS2* HS1 S663P (16 isolates). It is noteworthy that mutations at positions S663 and F659 tended to be associated with breakthrough infections in patients receiving echinocandin therapy [25,53]. In our case, the MIC results (later confirmed by *FKS* mutation results) were promptly available to clinicians, but given the patient's critical condition, the ensuing change of antifungal therapy was unsuccessful. Nevertheless, we acknowledge the importance of combining both antifungal susceptibility testing and *FKS* sequencing to predict therapeutic failure in candidemia patients treated with echinocandins [15]. This combination strategy would allow for encompassing cases of mutations occurring outside of HS *FKS* regions in echinocandin-resistant isolates [54], or cases of echinocandin-susceptible isolates carrying mutations in HS *FKS* regions in which the patients infected with such isolates show therapeutic failure following echinocandin treatment [55]. Ultimately, this strategy would ensure the choosing of an appropriate antifungal therapy in the clinic [15].

In conclusion, this case highlights that bacterial and fungal coinfections, including those associated with antimicrobial resistance, in COVID-19 may be a further challenge for both clinicians and microbiologists. In waiting for epidemiological studies to evaluate their frequency and impact, it is imperative to be vigilant for these coinfections when contemplating the outcome of COVID-19.

Author Contributions: Conceptualization, B.P., R.T., A.V., and M.F.; formal analysis, M.S.; investigation, R.T., A.V., and P.M.L.; resources, M.S.; data curation, G.D.A., E.D.C., and G.V.; writing—original draft preparation, B.P. and M.F.; writing—review and editing, R.T., A.V., G.D.A., and E.D.C.; supervision, M.S. and M.F. All authors have read and agreed to the published version of the manuscript.

Funding: This study received no external funding.

Acknowledgments: We wish to thank Franziska Lohmeyer for her English language assistance.

Conflicts of Interest: The authors declare no conflict of interest.

References

1. Zhu, N.; Zhang, D.; Wang, W.; Li, X.; Yang, B.; Song, J.; Zhao, X.; Huang, B.; Shi, W.; Lu, R.; et al. A novel coronavirus from patients with pneumonia in China, 2019. *N. Engl. J. Med.* **2020**, *382*, 727–733. [CrossRef]
2. World Health Organization. Coronavirus Disease (COVID-19). Situation Report—183. 21 July 2020. Available online: https://www.who.int/emergencies/diseases/novel-coronavirus-2019/situation-reports (accessed on 26 July 2020).
3. Ren, D.; Ren, C.; Yao, R.Q.; Feng, Y.W.; Yao, Y.M. Clinical features and development of sepsis in patients infected with SARS-CoV-2: A retrospective analysis of 150 cases outside Wuhan, China. *Intensiv. Care Med.* **2020**, *46*, 1630–1633. [CrossRef] [PubMed]
4. Rawson, T.M.; Moore, L.S.P.; Zhu, N.; Ranganathan, N.; Skolimowska, K.; Gilchrist, M.; Satta, G.; Cooke, G.; Holmes, A. Bacterial and Fungal Coinfection in Individuals with Coronavirus: A Rapid Review to Support COVID-19 Antimicrobial Prescribing. *Clin. Infect. Dis.* **2020**. [CrossRef] [PubMed]
5. Clancy, C.J.; Nguyen, M.H. COVID-19, superinfections and antimicrobial development: What can we expect? *Clin. Infect. Dis.* **2020**. [CrossRef]
6. Zhou, F.; Yu, T.; Du, R.; Fan, G.; Liu, Y.; Liu, Z.; Xiang, J.; Wang, Y.; Song, B.; Gu, X.; et al. Clinical course and risk factors for mortality of adult inpatients with COVID-19 in Wuhan, China: A retrospective cohort study. *Lancet* **2020**, *395*, 1054–1062. [CrossRef]
7. Ruan, Q.; Yang, K.; Wang, W.; Jiang, L.; Song, J. Clinical predictors of mortality due to COVID-19 based on an analysis of data of 150 patients from Wuhan, China. *Intensiv. Care Med.* **2020**, *46*, 846–848. [CrossRef] [PubMed]
8. Li, H.; Liu, L.; Zhang, D.; Xu, J.; Dai, H.; Tang, N.; Su, X.; Cao, B. SARS-CoV-2 and viral sepsis: Observations and hypotheses. *Lancet* **2020**, *395*, 1517–1520. [CrossRef]
9. Kox, M.; Frenzel, T.; Schouten, J.; van de Veerdonk, F.L.; Koenen, H.J.P.M.; Pickkers, P.; on behalf of the RCI-COVID-19 study group. COVID-19 patients exhibit less pronounced immune suppression compared with bacterial septic shock patients. *Crit. Care* **2020**, *24*, 263. [CrossRef]

10. Rodriguez-Morales, A.J.; Cardona-Ospina, J.A.; Gutiérrez-Ocampo, E.; Villamizar-Peña, R.; Holguin-Rivera, Y.; Escalera-Antezana, J.P.; Alvarado-Arnez, L.E.; Bonilla-Aldana, D.K.; Franco-Paredes, C.; Henao-Martinez, A.F.; et al. Clinical, laboratory and imaging features of COVID-19: A systematic review and meta-analysis. *Travel Med. Infect. Dis.* **2020**, *34*, 101623. [CrossRef]
11. Erener, S. Diabetes, infection risk and COVID-19. *Mol. Metab.* **2020**, *39*, 101044. [CrossRef]
12. Rao Kondapally Seshasai, S.; Kaptoge, S.; Thompson, A.; Di Angelantonio, E.; Gao, P.; Sarwar, N.; Whincup, P.H.; Mukamal, K.J.; Gillum, R.F.; Holme, I.; et al. Diabetes mellitus, fasting glucose, and risk of cause-specific death. *N. Engl. J. Med.* **2011**, *364*, 829–841. [PubMed]
13. Thaiss, C.A.; Levy, M.; Grosheva, I.; Zheng, D.; Soffer, E.; Blacher, E.; Braverman, S.; Tengeler, A.C.; Barak, O.; Elazar, M.; et al. Hyperglycemia drives intestinal barrier dysfunction and risk for enteric infection. *Science* **2018**, *359*, 1376–1383. [CrossRef] [PubMed]
14. Arastehfar, A.; Carvalho, A.; van de Veerdonk, F.L.; Jenks, J.D.; Koehler, P.; Krause, R.; Cornely, O.A.; Perlin, D.S.; Lass-Flörl, C.; Hoenigl, M. COVID-19 associated pulmonary aspergillosis (CAPA)—From immunology to treatment. *J. Fungi* **2020**, *6*, 91. [CrossRef] [PubMed]
15. Arastehfar, A.; Lass-Flörl, C.; Garcia-Rubio, R.; Daneshnia, F.; Ilkit, M.; Boekhout, T.; Gabaldon, T.; Perlin, D.S. The quiet and underappreciated rise of drug-resistant invasive fungal pathogens. *J. Fungi* **2020**, *6*, E138. [CrossRef]
16. Pfaller, M.A.; Diekema, D.J.; Turnidge, J.D.; Castanheira, M.; Jones, R.N. Twenty years of the SENTRY antifungal surveillance program: Results for *Candida* species from 1997–2016. *Open Forum Infect. Dis.* **2019**, *6*, S79–S94. [CrossRef]
17. Arastehfar, A.; Yazdanpanah, S.; Bakhtiari, M.; Fang, W.; Pan, W.; Mahmoudi, S.; Pakshir, K.; Daneshnia, F.; Boekhout, T.; Ilkit, M.; et al. Epidemiology of candidemia in Shiraz, southern Iran: A prospective multicenter study (2016–2018). *Med. Mycol.* **2020**, myaa059. [CrossRef]
18. Corman, V.M.; Landt, O.; Kaiser, M.; Molenkamp, R.; Meijer, A.; Chu, D.K.; Bleicker, T.; Brünink, S.; Schneider, J.; Schmidt, M.L.; et al. Detection of 2019 novel coronavirus (2019-nCoV) by real-time RT-PCR. *Euro Surveill.* **2020**, *25*, 2000045. [CrossRef]
19. World Health Organization. Laboratory Testing for Coronavirus Disease (COVID-19) in Suspected Human Cases: Interim Guidance. 2020. Available online: https://apps.who.int/iris/bitstream/handle/10665/331501/WHO-COVID-19-laboratory-2020.5-eng.pdf?sequence=1&isAllowed=y (accessed on 26 July 2020).
20. De Carolis, E.; Vella, A.; Vaccaro, L.; Torelli, R.; Posteraro, P.; Ricciardi, W.; Sanguinetti, M.; Posteraro, B. Development and validation of an in-house database for matrix-assisted laser desorption ionization-time of flight mass spectrometry-based yeast identification using a fast protein extraction procedure. *J. Clin. Microbiol.* **2014**, *52*, 1453–1458. [CrossRef]
21. Clinical and Laboratory Standards Institute. *Reference Method for Broth Dilution Antifungal Susceptibility Testing of Yeasts*; Approved Standard CLSI Document M27-A3; Clinical and Laboratory Standards Institute: Wayne, PA, USA, 2008.
22. Clinical and Laboratory Standards Institute. *Performance Standards for Antifungal susceptibility Testing of Yeasts*; Approved standard M60; Clinical and Laboratory Standards Institute: Wayne, PA, USA, 2017.
23. Clinical and Laboratory Standards Institute. *Epidemiological Cutoff Values for Antifungal Susceptibility Testing*; CLSI supplement M59; Clinical and Laboratory Standards Institute: Wayne, PA, USA, 2018.
24. Castanheira, M.; Woosley, L.N.; Diekema, D.J.; Messer, S.A.; Jones, R.N.; Pfaller, M.A. Low prevalence of *fks1* hot spot 1 mutations in a worldwide collection of *Candida* strains. *Antimicrob. Agents Chemother.* **2010**, *54*, 2655–2659. [CrossRef]
25. Alexander, B.D.; Johnson, M.D.; Pfeiffer, C.D.; Jiménez-Ortigosa, C.; Catania, J.; Booker, R.; Castanheira, M.; Messer, S.A.; Perlin, D.S.; Pfaller, M.A. Increasing echinocandin resistance in *Candida glabrata*: Clinical failure correlates with presence of *FKS* mutations and elevated minimum inhibitory concentrations. *Clin. Infect. Dis.* **2013**, *56*, 1724–1732. [CrossRef]
26. Wright, W.F.; Bejou, N.; Shields, R.K.; Marr, K.; McCarty, T.P.; Pappas, P.G. Amphotericin B induction with voriconazole consolidation as salvage therapy for *FKS*-associated echinocandin resistance in *Candida glabrata* septic arthritis and osteomyelitis. *Antimicrob. Agents Chemother.* **2019**, *63*, e00512–e00519. [CrossRef] [PubMed]

27. Yang, J.; Zheng, Y.; Gou, X.; Pu, K.; Chen, Z.; Guo, Q.; Ji, R.; Wang, H.; Wang, Y.; Zhou, Y. Prevalence of comorbidities and its effects in patients infected with SARS-CoV-2: A systematic review and meta-analysis. *Int. J. Infect. Dis.* **2020**, *94*, 91–95. [CrossRef] [PubMed]
28. Zhu, L.; She, Z.G.; Cheng, X.; Qin, J.J.; Zhang, X.J.; Cai, J.; Lei, F.; Wang, H.; Xie, J.; Wang, W.; et al. Association of blood glucose control and outcomes in patients with covid-19 and pre-existing type 2 diabetes. *Cell Metab.* **2020**, *31*, 1068–1077. [CrossRef] [PubMed]
29. Gangneux, J.P.; Bougnoux, M.E.; Dannaoui, E.; Cornet, M.; Zahar, J.R. Invasive fungal diseases during COVID-19: We should be prepared. *J. Mycol. Med.* **2020**, *30*, 100971. [CrossRef]
30. Tay, M.Z.; Poh, C.M.; Rénia, L.; MacAry, P.A.; Ng, L.F.P. The trinity of COVID-19: Immunity, inflammation and intervention. *Nat. Rev. Immunol.* **2020**, *20*, 363–374. [CrossRef]
31. Chen, N.; Zhou, M.; Dong, X.; Qu, J.; Gong, F.; Han, Y.; Qiu, Y.; Wang, J.; Liu, Y.; Wei, Y.; et al. Epidemiological and clinical characteristics of 99 cases of 2019 novel coronavirus pneumonia in Wuhan, China: A descriptive study. *Lancet* **2020**, *395*, 507–513. [CrossRef]
32. Iacob, S.; Iacob, D.G. Infectious threats, the intestinal barrier, and its Trojan horse: Dysbiosis. *Front. Microbiol.* **2019**, *10*, 1676. [CrossRef]
33. Zhai, B.; Ola, M.; Rolling, T.; Tosini, N.L.; Joshowitz, S.; Littmann, E.R.; Amoretti, L.A.; Fontana, E.; Wright, R.J.; Miranda, E.; et al. High-resolution mycobiota analysis reveals dynamic intestinal translocation preceding invasive candidiasis. *Nat. Med.* **2020**, *26*, 59–64. [CrossRef]
34. Rodrigues, C.F.; Silva, S.; Henriques, M. *Candida glabrata*: A review of its features and resistance. *Eur. J. Clin. Microbiol. Infect. Dis.* **2014**, *33*, 673–688. [CrossRef]
35. McCarty, T.P.; Lockhart, S.R.; Moser, S.A.; Whiddon, J.; Zurko, J.; Pham, C.D.; Pappas, P.G. Echinocandin resistance among *Candida* isolates at an academic medical centre 2005-15: Analysis of trends and outcomes. *J. Antimicrob. Chemother.* **2018**, *73*, 1677–1680. [CrossRef]
36. Perlin, D.S.; Rautemaa-Richardson, R.; Alastruey-Izquierdo, A. The global problem of antifungal resistance: Prevalence, mechanisms, and management. *Lancet Infect. Dis.* **2017**, *17*, e383–e392. [CrossRef]
37. Pappas, P.G.; Kauffman, C.A.; Andes, D.R.; Clancy, C.J.; Marr, K.A.; Ostrosky-Zeichner, L.; Reboli, A.C.; Schuster, M.G.; Vazquez, J.A.; Walsh, T.J.; et al. Clinical practice guideline for the management of candidiasis: 2016 update by the Infectious Diseases Society of America. *Clin. Infect. Dis.* **2016**, *62*, e1–e50. [CrossRef] [PubMed]
38. Ostrosky-Zeichner, L.; Al-Obaidi, M. Invasive fungal infections in the intensive care unit. *Infect. Dis. Clin. N. Am.* **2017**, *31*, 475–487. [CrossRef]
39. Agnelli, C.; Guinea, J.; Valerio, M.; Escribano, P.; Bouza, E.; Muñoz, P. Infectious endocarditis caused by *Candida glabrata*: Evidence of in vivo development of echinocandin resistance. *Rev. Esp. Quimioter.* **2019**, *32*, 395–397. [PubMed]
40. Lewis, J.S., II; Wiederhold, N.P.; Wickes, B.L.; Patterson, T.F.; Jorgensen, J.H. Rapid emergence of echinocandin resistance in *Candida glabrata* resulting in clinical and microbiologic failure. *Antimicrob. Agents Chemother.* **2013**, *57*, 4559–4561. [CrossRef]
41. Shields, R.K.; Nguyen, M.H.; Press, E.G.; Updike, C.L.; Clancy, C.J. Caspofungin MICs correlate with treatment outcomes among patients with *Candida glabrata* invasive candidiasis and prior echinocandin exposure. *Antimicrob. Agents Chemother.* **2013**, *57*, 3528–3535. [CrossRef] [PubMed]
42. Shields, R.K.; Nguyen, M.H.; Press, E.G.; Clancy, C.J. Abdominal candidiasis is a hidden reservoir of echinocandin resistance. *Antimicrob. Agents Chemother.* **2014**, *58*, 7601–7605. [CrossRef]
43. Healey, K.R.; Nagasaki, Y.; Zimmerman, M.; Kordalewska, M.; Park, S.; Zhao, Y.; Perlin, D.S. The gastrointestinal tract is a major source of echinocandin drug resistance in a murine model of *Candida glabrata* colonization and systemic dissemination. *Antimicrob. Agents Chemother.* **2017**, *61*, e01412–e01417. [CrossRef]
44. Bordallo-Cardona, M.Á.; Escribano, P.; de la Pedrosa, E.G.; Marcos-Zambrano, L.J.; Cantón, R.; Bouza, E.; Guinea, J. In vitro exposure to increasing micafungin concentrations easily promotes echinocandin resistance in *Candida glabrata* isolates. *Antimicrob. Agents Chemother.* **2017**, *61*, e01542-16. [CrossRef]
45. Shields, R.K.; Kline, E.G.; Healey, K.R.; Kordalewska, M.; Perlin, D.S.; Nguyen, M.H.; Clancy, C.J. Spontaneous mutational frequency and *FKS* mutation rates vary by echinocandin agent against *Candida glabrata*. *Antimicrob. Agents Chemother.* **2018**, *63*, e01692-18. [CrossRef]

46. Healey, K.R.; Katiyar, S.K.; Castanheira, M.; Pfaller, M.A.; Edlind, T.D. *Candida glabrata* mutants demonstrating paradoxical reduced caspofungin susceptibility but increased micafungin susceptibility. *Antimicrob. Agents Chemother.* **2011**, *55*, 3947–3949. [CrossRef] [PubMed]
47. Lee, K.K.; Maccallum, D.M.; Jacobsen, M.D.; Walker, L.A.; Odds, F.C.; Gow, N.A.; Munro, C.A. Elevated cell wall chitin in *Candida albicans* confers echinocandin resistance in vivo. *Antimicrob. Agents Chemother.* **2012**, *56*, 208–217. [CrossRef] [PubMed]
48. Katiyar, S.K.; Alastruey-Izquierdo, A.; Healey, K.R.; Johnson, M.E.; Perlin, D.S.; Edlind, T.D. Fks1 and Fks2 are functionally redundant but differentially regulated in *Candida glabrata*: Implications for echinocandin resistance. *Antimicrob. Agents Chemother.* **2012**, *56*, 6304–6309. [CrossRef] [PubMed]
49. Arendrup, M.C.; Perlin, D.S. Echinocandin resistance: An emerging clinical problem? *Curr. Opin. Infect. Dis.* **2014**, *27*, 484–492. [CrossRef]
50. Bordallo-Cardona, M.Á.; Sánchez-Carrillo, C.; Bouza, E.; Muñoz, P.; Escribano, P.; Guinea, J. Detection of echinocandin-resistant *Candida glabrata* in blood cultures spiked with different percentages of *FKS2* mutants. *Antimicrob. Agents Chemother.* **2019**, *63*, e02004–e02018.
51. De Angelis, G.; Menchinelli, G.; Torelli, R.; De Carolis, E.; Posteraro, P.; Sanguinetti, M.; Posteraro, B. Different detection capabilities by mycological media for *Candida* isolates from mono- or dual-species cultures. *PLoS ONE* **2020**, *15*, e0226467. [CrossRef]
52. Garcia-Effron, G.; Lee, S.; Park, S.; Cleary, J.D.; Perlin, D.S. Effect of *Candida glabrata FKS1* and *FKS2* mutations on echinocandin sensitivity and kinetics of 1,3-beta-D-glucan synthase: Implication for the existing susceptibility breakpoint. *Antimicrob. Agents Chemother.* **2009**, *53*, 3690–3699. [CrossRef]
53. Shields, R.K.; Nguyen, M.H.; Press, E.G.; Kwa, A.L.; Cheng, S.; Du, C.; Clancy, C.J. The presence of an *FKS* mutation rather than MIC is an independent risk factor for failure of echinocandin therapy among patients with invasive candidiasis due to *Candida glabrata*. *Antimicrob. Agents Chemother.* **2012**, *56*, 4862–4869. [CrossRef]
54. Hou, X.; Healey, K.R.; Shor, E.; Kordalewska, M.; Ortigosa, C.J.; Paderu, P.; Xiao, M.; Wang, H.; Zhao, Y.; Lin, L.Y.; et al. Novel *FKS1* and *FKS2* modifications in a high-level echinocandin resistant clinical isolate of *Candida glabrata*. *Emerg. Microbes Infect.* **2019**, *8*, 1619–1625. [CrossRef]
55. Arastehfar, A.; Daneshnia, F.; Salehi, M.; Yaşar, M.; Hoşbul, T.; Ilkit, M.; Pan, W.; Hagen, F.; Arslan, N.; Türk-Dağı, H.; et al. Low level of antifungal resistance of *Candida glabrata* blood isolates in Turkey: Fluconazole minimum inhibitory concentration and *FKS* mutations can predict therapeutic failure. *Mycoses* **2020**, *63*, 911–920. [CrossRef]

Journal of
Fungi

MDPI

Case Report

Bloodstream Infection by *Saccharomyces cerevisiae* in Two COVID-19 Patients after Receiving Supplementation of *Saccharomyces* in the ICU

Ioannis Ventoulis [1], Theopisti Sarmourli [2], Pinelopi Amoiridou [1], Paraskevi Mantzana [3], Maria Exindari [2], Georgia Gioula [2] and Timoleon-Achilleas Vyzantiadis [2,*]

1 Intensive Care Unit, "Bodossakio" General Hospital of Ptolemaida, 50200 Ptolemaida, Greece; ventoulis@hotmail.com (I.V.); pamoirid@yahoo.gr (P.A.)

2 Department of Microbiology, Medical School, Aristotle University of Thessaloniki, 54124 Thessaloniki, Greece; p.sarmourli@gmail.com (T.S.); mexidari@auth.gr (M.E.); ggioula@med.auth.gr (G.G.)

3 Department of Microbiology, AHEPA Hospital, Aristotle University of Thessaloniki, 54636 Thessaloniki, Greece; vimantzana@gmail.com

* Correspondence: tavyz@auth.gr; Tel.: +30-2310-999027

Received: 10 June 2020; Accepted: 29 June 2020; Published: 30 June 2020

Abstract: Co-infections have an unknown impact on the morbidity and mortality of the new clinical syndrome called coronavirus disease 2019 (COVID-19). The syndrome is caused by the new pandemic coronavirus SARS-CoV-2 and it is probably connected with severe traces in the elements of the immune system. Apart from possible *Aspergillus* infections, particularly in patients with acute respiratory distress syndrome (ARDS), other fungal infections could occur, probably more easily, due to the immunological dysregulation and the critical condition of these patients. Probiotic preparations of *Saccharomyces* are broadly used for the prevention of antibiotic-associated complications, especially in the intensive care units (ICU). On the other hand, *Saccharomyces* organisms are reported as agents of invasive infection in immunocompromised or critically ill patients. We report two cases of bloodstream infection by *Saccharomyces* in two patients hospitalised in the ICU, due to severe COVID-19, after *Saccharomyces* supplementation.

Keywords: COVID-19; fungaemia; *Saccharomyces*; co-infections

1. Introduction

The new pandemic caused by the coronavirus SARS-CoV-2 has evolved as a major health threat and has been connected to a big number of deaths worldwide, while the future spread of the disease is more or less unknown.

While it is already known that patients with co-morbidities and underlying diseases present poorer clinical outcomes [1], the frequency of co-infections and their impact is still understudied [2].

There are common risk factors, such as hospitalisation in the intensive care unit (ICU), chronic respiratory diseases, corticosteroid therapy or intubation and mechanical ventilation [2] that could serve as the field for a co-infection by SARS-CoV-2 and an invasive fungus. As in cases of severe influenza and the known co-morbidity with invasive pulmonary aspergillosis [3,4], cases of patients hospitalised in the ICU for coronavirus disease 2019 (COVID-19) with acute respiratory distress syndrome (ARDS), who suffered a co-infection by *Aspergillus*, have already been reported [5–8].

Saccharomyces cerevisiae has been a well-known and emerging agent of invasive fungal infection since the 1990s in immunocompromised or critically ill patients [9]. While it is a known coloniser or even as part of the normal flora [10] and it is often used in probiotic preparations for the prevention or treatment of various diarrheal disorders [11], it can cause several types of deep infections, most importantly fungaemia [9].

We report two cases of critically ill patients who had to be hospitalised in the ICU due to COVID-19, received *Saccharomyces cerevisiae* supplementation because of diarrhea, and subsequently developed a *Saccharomyces cerevisiae* bloodstream infection. Informed consent was acquired from both patients with opt out possibility.

2. Case Reports

They concern two male patients, 76 and 73 years old, with no other underlying diseases apart from regulated arterial hypertension (both of them) and diabetes (the second). The first one was also an ex-smoker.

Both patients presented fever, dyspnea and hypoxia, while the second also had a nonproductive cough. They were admitted for hospitalisation by different departments of internal medicine. In two days' time, due to the worsening of their clinical condition and the concomitant development of ARDS, they had to be intubated and subsequently transferred to the ICU.

Meanwhile, the molecular testing for SARS-CoV-2 was found positive in both patients' upper and lower respiratory specimens by the use of real time RT-PCR methods (diagnostic detection protocol for 2019-nCoV, Charité, Berlin, via EVAg and/or VIASURE SARS-CoV-2 detection kit, CerTest Biotec, SL, Zaragoza, Spain). The first patient was found positive again ten and fifteen days later, while he became negative almost twenty-five days later. The second patient was positive when retested on the fifteenth day and negative twenty days later.

During their stay at the ICU they had several successive positive blood cultures for *Staphylococcus hominis* and *Acinetobacter baumannii* first and *Staphylococcus epidermidis* and *Acinetobacter baumannii* second. Moreover, *Acinetobacter baumannii* and *Pseudomonas aeruginosa* were isolated from the cultures of their bronchial secretions.

The first patient, from the day of his admission in the ICU and for ten days thereafter, had a positive blood culture for *Staphylococcus hominis* and, at day 26, for *Acinetobacter baumannii*, which continued even up to day 45. Meanwhile, at day 11, he presented a positive bronchial culture for *Pseudomonas aeruginosa* and, from day 26 and thereafter, for *Acinetobacter baumannii*.

The second patient had a positive blood culture at day 10 by *Acinetobacter baumannii* and at day 15 by *Staphylococcus epidermidis*. The presence of *Acinetobacter baumannii* relapsed at day 18, while all blood cultures became negative at day 30. He also had positive bronchial cultures for *Acinetobacter baumannii* between days 10 and 15 and again from day 18 to day 30.

For all the aforementioned blood and bronchial infections, the two patients received empirical, as well as documented (by culture and sensitivity testing), treatment with several antibiotics, such as piperacillin–tazobactam, moxifloxacin, linezolid, azithromycin, meropenem, colistin, daptomycin and tigecycline. The sequence of the relevant antimicrobials is seen in Table 1. In addition to that, both patients were under treatment with oseltamivir and hydroxychloroquine.

Moreover, the two patients developed a gradual worsening of their renal function and had to undergo several sessions of haemodialysis. The decrease in the kidney capacity could be attributed to both the accumulative nephrotoxicity of several of the antimicrobials, as well as to the COVID-19 itself [12].

Both patients developed diarrhea and were prophylactically treated with Ultra-Levure (preparation of *Saccharomyces cerevisiae* (*boulardii*)) at 250 to 500 mg/day.

The first patient, thirty-five days after his admission at the ICU, while febrile (38–38.5 °C), suffered a bloodstream infection by *Saccharomyces cerevisiae* (Table 1). The same happened with the second patient, fifteen days after his admission to the ICU. Both episodes were possibly related to the use of Ultra-Levure, as they occurred four days after its initiation in the first case and six days in the second one. Initially and before the fungal identification and the sensitivity testing, they were treated with anidulafungin and afterwards with fluconazole. Blood cultures became negative three to four days later, while the treatment with fluconazole continued for fourteen days. Blood cultures were taken daily, from the first positive up to the first negative result, while patients remained fungaemic in the first two days of their antifungal treatment.

Table 1. Antimicrobials, duration of treatment, Sepsis-Related Organ Failure Assessment scores (SOFA scores), laboratory values and fever on indicative days.

Patient	***Saccharomyces* in Blood Culture**					
	Day 1	Day 11	Day 26	Day 35	Day 45	
Patient 1	Piperacillin-tazobactam and Linezolid (14 days) Moxifloxacin (10 days) Azithromycin (5 days)	Meropenem (14 days)	Colistin and Tigecycline (21 days)	Anidulafungin (10 days)	Fluconazole (14 days)	
	T: 38.5 °C WBC: 7500/mL Neut.: 92% CRP: 39.5 SOFA: 9			T: 38 °C WBC: 9200/mL Neut.: 50% CRP: 21.6 PCT: 1.04 SOFA: 3	T: 37.5 °C WBC: 9300/mL Neut.: 58% CRP: 8.6 PCT: 0.66 SOFA: 5	
	***Saccharomyces* in Blood Culture**					
	Day 1	Day 10	Day 15	Day 18	Day 23	Day 30
Patient 2	Piperacillin-tazobactam (12 days) Linezolid (14 days) Moxifloxacin (10 days) Azithromycin (3 days)	Meropenem (7 days) Colistin (21 days)	Anidulafungin (7 days) Daptomycin (7 days)	Anidulafungin Tigecycline (7 days)	Fluconazole (14 days) Tigecycline Linezolid (8 days)	
	T: 39.0 °C WBC: 8900/mL Neut.: 93% CRP: 26.54 PCT: 0.9 SOFA: 6		T: 38.3 °C WBC: 17500/mL Neut.: 82% CRP: 13.15 PCT: 1.15 SOFA: 9		SOFA: 9	T: 37.0 °C WBC: 7600/mL Neut.: 72% CRP: 6.0 PCT: 0.9 SOFA: 4

Temperature (T), white blood cell count (WBC), neutrophils (Neut.), C-reactive protein (CRP, 0–0.5 mg/dL), procalcitonin (PCT, 0–0.5 ng/mL), Sepsis-Related Organ Failure Assessment score (SOFA score).

After the incubation of the blood cultures, positive direct microscopy and inoculation on Sabouraud dextrose agar with chloramphenicol 0.05% (Conda Pronadisa, Madrid, Spain) and malt extract agar (Sigma-Aldrich Co., St. Louis, MO, USA) at 30 °C and 35 °C, the use of germ tube testing and CHROMagar Candida (Paris, France) and biochemical testing by API ID 32C (bioMérieux SA, Marcy l' Etoile, France), the two strains were phenotypically identified as *Saccharomyces cerevisiae*.

Further on, both identifications were molecularly confirmed by the amplification and sequencing of the internal transcribed spacer 1 (ITS1) region of the fungal ribosomal DNA (Gen Bank Accession Numbers: MT527544 and MT522376). Both sequences presented a 100% alignment between each other, as well as with the sequence of the strain used in the specific preparation of Ultra-Levure, providing arguments for the genetic relatedness and similarity of all three of them.

A sensitivity testing was attempted by ATB™ Fungus 3 (bioMérieux SA, Marcy l' Etoile, France) for amphotericin B, flucytosine, fluconazole, itraconazole and voriconazole and MIC (minimum inhibitory concentration) Test Strips (Liofilchem srl, Roseto degli Abruzzi, Italy) for posaconazole and anidulafungin, although there are possible difficulties concerning the growth of *Saccahromyces* and, mainly, *boulardii* on RPMI agar [9]. The growth on RPMI agar was slightly delayed, but after two days of incubation there was a slight, yet adequate, growth that permitted the read.

The MICs for the first isolate were 4 μg/mL for flucytosine, 1.0 μg/mL for amphotericin-B, 0.5 μg/mL for itraconazole, 4.0 μg/mL for fluconazole, 0.125 μg/mL for voriconazole, 0.032 μg/mL for posaconazole and 0.047 μg/mL for anidulafungin, while, for the second one, they were 4 μg/mL for flucytosine,

0.5 μg/mL for amphotericin-B, 0.5 μg/mL for itraconazole, 4.0 μg/mL for fluconazole, 0.125 μg/mL for voriconazole, 0.064 μg/mL for posaconazole and 0.002 μg/mL for anidulafungin. Although there are not defined clinical breakpoints for *Saccharomyces*, the above results indicate a probable in vitro sensitivity to flucytosine, amphotericin-B, fluconazole, voriconazole, posaconazole and anidulafungin.

In both patients, no fungal presence was found in any of the bronchial cultures.

Gradually, both patients showed clinical improvement and were transferred again to the department of internal medicine of the hospital. The first patient, after almost eighty days of hospitalisation, was discharged from the hospital, while the second had to be transferred to a regional teaching hospital due to complications with his tracheostomy.

3. The ICU

Both described patients were hospitalised in a small and relatively new intensive care unit with four beds. Due to the outbreak of COVID-19, two more beds, exclusively for these patients, were added. These beds were separated from the rest of the ICU and from one another, while separate nursing staff were provided for each COVID-19 patient. Moreover, all necessary, very strict measures were taken in order to maintain "sterile" conditions between the patients.

According to the experience of the medical staff of the unit and the well-recorded data, no case of fungaemia due to *Saccharomyces* had occurred for at least the last four years in this ICU, despite the fact that it was a long lasting and common practice to use preparations of the fungus for the prophylaxis of patients under antibiotics and concomitant diarrhea. During the last four years, almost eighty patients per year (320 patients in total) were to in this specific ICU and at least half of them were under prophylactic preparations of *Saccharomyces*. This was the first time that such a fungaemia occurred and only during the hospitalisation of these first two COVID patients.

4. Discussion

Apart from the devastating consequences of SARS-CoV-2 on the respiratory function, there are also pronounced effects on the absolute numbers of lymphocytes, leading to lymphopenia and an increase in several cytokines and inflammatory markers [13–15]. Lymphopenia could be attributed to the virus directly or the white blood cell redistribution, as the T_{CD8} cells have a major role in the clearing of the virus from the pulmonary tissue. However, these cells can be relatively dysfunctional due to the highly produced epithelial cytokines and the impairment of their function could affect the function of dendritic cells and macrophages [16–18]. All of the above suggest immune dysfunction and, at least, a host immune imbalance to several extents [19].

The administration of probiotic preparations containing live yeasts, like *Saccharomyces*, may pose a high risk to patients suffering from immune deficiencies due to malignancies or immunosuppressive treatment. Moreover, oral mucositis or ulcers may lead to yeast translocation into the bloodstream of such patients [20,21]. Central venous catheters in critically ill patients could serve as the site of entry due to hand transmission [22,23], although the main portal of entry for invasive infections by *Saccharomyces cerevisiae* is supposed to be digestive [9]. Further on, nosocomial acquisition may occur from patients hospitalised in the same unit [24]. Yeasts persist on room surfaces and at distances of 1 m after the opening of the capsule for administration through the nasogastric tube, while they can also be detected on the hands of healthcare workers [25].

Saccharomyces boulardii, which is used in commercial probiotic preparations is considered to be an invalid taxon and either a subtype or a variety of *Saccharomyces cerevisiae* [9,26,27], in fact identical to a particular strain of the latter [28]. Fungaemia by *S. boulardii*, after probiotic use, is more often seen in critically ill patients in the ICU rather than in typical immunodeficient patients [9,20,28]. However, this could be attributed to the prophylactic use of antifungals as routine treatment in immunocompromised, such as oncohaematological, patients [20].

In the described cases, it is interesting that, although the probiotic preparations of *Saccharomyces cerevisiae/boulardii* were used for many years as protective agents in this specific ICU and even during the same period of hospitalisation of other patients, only the two specific patients with COVID-19 presented a bloodstream infection. The fact that they were completely separated from one another and the other patients of the ICU and were treated by separate nursing staff, with all the recommended precautions for the avoidance of SARS-CoV-2 transmission, extremely reduces the chances of being contaminated by manipulations or acquisition from other patients or personnel and makes a connection to the probiotic preparations more possible.

In addition, the fact that both fungaemias occurred four to six days after the initiation of Ultra-Levure makes even more possible the connection of the infection to the use of the specific preparation and the concomitant fungal translocation from the gastrointestinal tract to the bloodstream.

Yeast overgrowth and gastrointestinal (GI) leakage, caused by either direct or indirect gastrointestinal injury, could be important pathogenic factors for invasive mycoses. Among other factors, intestinal surgery, haemodialysis, intensive chemotherapy and sepsis could play important roles in the aforementioned GI leakage. Moreover, there are indications that the occurrence of fungal translocation through mucosal barrier damage, as indirectly calculated by the measurement of serum (1→3) β-D-glucan, is correlated to Sepsis-Related Organ Failure Assessment score (SOFA score) and the gravity of the disease in terms of septic shock [29,30].

It is reported that the sequencing of the ITS region of the fungal ribosomal DNA cannot possibly discriminate *S. boulardii* from some *S. cerevisiae* strains [9,31]. However, herein, the results of a 100% alignment between the ITS1 sequences of the patients' strains and the strain used in the specific preparation of Ultra-Levure, combined with the clinical data, show a good similarity and provide arguments for the genetic relatedness of all three of them.

Although further data and observations are needed, the occurrence of the described cases of two patients suffering from severe COVID-19, with long periods of hospitalisation in the ICU and concomitant bloodstream infection by *Saccharomyces cerevisae*, indicates the need for cautious use of the relevant probiotic preparations in COVID-19 patients.

Author Contributions: I.V. and P.A. were the responsible intensivists for all the clinical care and treatment of the two patients. They provided all the necessary clinical information. T.S. together with T.-A.V. did the laboratory identification, the sensitivity testing and the molecular analysis of the fungal strains. P.M. did the culture and initial identification of one of the strains, while M.E. and G.G. were the responsible for the COVID-19 testing. T.-A.V. being responsible of the mycology laboratory initiated the study, wrote the draft version, reviewed and edited the whole study through the preparation period and till the finalisation of the manuscript. All authors have read and agreed to the published version of the manuscript.

Funding: This research received no external funding.

Conflicts of Interest: The authors declare no conflict of interest.

References

1. Guan, W.J.; Liang, W.H.; Zhao, Y.; Liang, H.R.; Chen, Z.S.; Li, Y.M.; Liu, X.Q.; Chen, R.C.; Tang, C.L.; Wang, T.; et al. Comorbidity and its impact on 1590 patients with COVID-19 in China: A Nationwide Analysis. *Eur. Respir. J.* **2020**, *55*, 2000547. [CrossRef]
2. Gangneux, J.P.; Bougnoux, M.E.; Cornet, M.; Zahar, J.R. Invasive fungal disease during COVID-19: We should be prepared. *J. Mycol. Med.* **2020**, *30*, 100971. [CrossRef]
3. European Centre for Disease Prevention and Control. *Influenza-Associated Invasive Pulmonary Aspergillosis, Europe—30 November 2018*; ECDC: Stockh, Sweden, 2018.
4. Koehler, P.; Bassetti, M.; Kochanek, M.; Shimabukuro-Vornhagen, A.; Cornely, O.A. Intensive Care Management of Influenza-Associated Pulmonary Aspergillosis. *Clin. Microbiol. Infect.* **2019**, *25*, 1501–1509. [CrossRef]
5. Yang, X.; Yu, Y.; Xu, J.; Shu, H.; Xia, J.; Liu, H.; Wu, Y.; Zhang, L.; Yu, Z.; Fang, M.; et al. Clinical course and outcomes of critically ill patients with SARS-CoV-2 pneumonia in Wuhan, China: A single centered, retrospective, observational study. *Lancet Respir. Med.* **2020**, *8*, 475–481. [CrossRef]
6. Koehler, P.; Cornely, O.A.; Böttiger, B.W.; Dusse, F.; Eichenauer, D.A.; Fuchs, F.; Hallek, M.; Jung, N.; Klein, F.; Persigehl, T.; et al. COVID-19 associated pulmonary aspergillosis. *Mycoses* **2020**, *63*, 528–534. [CrossRef]

7. Alanio, A.; Dellière, S.; Fodil, S.; Bretagne, S.; Mégarbane, B. Prevalence of putative invasive pulmonary aspergillosis in critically ill patients with COVID-19. *Lancet Respir. Med.* **2020**, *8*, e48–e49. [CrossRef]
8. Prattes, J.; Valentin, T.; Hoenigl, M.; Talakic, E.; Reisinger, A.C.; Eller, P. Invasive Pulmonary Aspergillosis Complicating COVID-19 in the ICU- A Case Report. *Med. Mycol. Case Rep.* **2020**. [CrossRef]
9. Enache-Angoulvant, A.; Hennequin, C. Invasive Saccharomyces Infection: A Comprehensive Review. *Clin. Infect. Dis.* **2005**, *41*, 1559–1568. [CrossRef] [PubMed]
10. Salonen, J.H.; Richardson, M.D.; Gallacher, K.; Issakainen, J.; Helenius, H.; Lehtonen, O.P.; Nikoskelainen, J. Fungal colonization of haematological patients receiving cytotoxic chemotherapy: Emergence of azole-resistant *Saccharomyces cerevisiae*. *J. Hosp. Infect.* **2000**, *45*, 293–301. [CrossRef] [PubMed]
11. Marteau, P.R.; de Vrese, M.; Cellier, C.J.; Schrezenmeir, J. Protection from gastrointestinal disease with the use of probiotics. *Am. J. Clin. Nutr.* **2001**, *73*, 430S–436S. [CrossRef] [PubMed]
12. Batlle, D.; Soler, M.J.; Sparks, M.A.; Hiremath, S.; South, A.M.; Welling, P.A.; Swaminathan, S.; COVID-19 and ACE2 in Cardiovascular, Lung, and Kidney Working Group. Acute Kidney Injury in COVID-19: Emerging Evidence of a Distinct Pathophysiology. *J. Am. Soc. Nephrol.* **2020**. [CrossRef] [PubMed]
13. He, F.; Deng, Y.; Li, W. Coronavirus disease 2019 (COVID-19): What we know? *J. Med. Virol.* **2020**, *92*, 719–725. [CrossRef]
14. Chen, G.; Wu, D.; Guo, W.; Cao, Y.; Huang, D.; Wang, H.; Wang, T.; Zhang, X.; Chen, H.; Yu, H.; et al. Clinical and immunologic features in severe and moderate Coronavirus disease 2019. *J. Clin. Investig.* **2020**, *130*, 2620–2629. [CrossRef]
15. He, L.; Ding, Y.; Zhang, Q.; Che, X.; He, Y.; Shen, H.; Wang, H.; Li, Z.; Zhao, L.; Geng, J.; et al. Expression of elevated levels of pro-inflammatory cytokines in SARS-CoV-infected ACE2+ cells in SARS patients: Relation to the acute lung injury and pathogenesis of SARS. *J. Pathol.* **2006**, *210*, 288–297. [CrossRef] [PubMed]
16. Yoshikawa, T.; Hill, T.; Li, K.; Peters, C.J.; Tseng, C.-T.K. Severe Acute Respiratory Syndrome (SARS) coronavirus-induced lung epithelial cytokines exacerbate sars pathogenesis by modulating intrinsic functions of monocyte-derived macrophages and dendritic cells. *J. Virol.* **2009**, *83*, 3039–3048. [CrossRef]
17. Xu, X.; Gao, X. Immunological responses against SARS-coronavirus infection in humans. *Cell Mol. Immunol.* **2004**, *1*, 119–122. [PubMed]
18. Li, G.; Fan, Y.; Lai, Y.; Han, T.; Li, Z.; Zhou, P.; Pan, P.; Wang, W.; Hu, D.; Liu, X.; et al. Coronavirus infections and immune responses. *J. Med. Virol.* **2020**, *92*, 424–432. [CrossRef]
19. Sarzi-Puttini, P.; Giorgi, V.; Sirotti, S.; Marotto, D.; Ardizzone, S.; Rizzardini, G.; Antinori, S.; Galli, M. COVID-19, cytokines and immunosuppression: What can we learn from severe acute respiratory syndrome? *Clin. Exp. Rheumatol.* **2020**, *38*, 337–342.
20. Sulik-Tyszka, B.; Snarski, E.; Niedźwiedzka, M.; Augustyniak, M.; Myhre, T.N.; Kacprzyk, A.; Swoboda-Kopeć, E.; Roszkowska, M.; Dwilewicz-Trojaczek, J.; Jędrzejczak, W.W.; et al. Experience with *Saccharomyces boulardii* Probiotic in Oncohaematological Patients. *Probiotics Antimicrob. Proteins* **2018**, *10*, 350–355. [CrossRef]
21. Tomblyn, M.; Chiller, T.; Einsele, H.; Gress, R.; Sepkowitz, K.; Storek, J.; Wingard, J.R.; Young, J.-A.H.; Boeckh, M.J.; Center for International Blood and Marrow Research; et al. Guidelines for preventing infectious complications among hematopoietic cell transplantation recipients: A global perspective. *Biol. Blood Marrow Transplant.* **2009**, *15*, 1143–1238. [CrossRef]
22. Lherm, T.; Monet, C.; Nougiere, B.; Soulier, M.; Larbi, D.; le Gall, C.; Caen, D.; Malbrunot, C. Seven cases of fungemia with *Saccharomyces boulardii* in critically ill patients. *Intensive Care Med.* **2002**, *28*, 797–801. [CrossRef] [PubMed]
23. Cassone, M.; Serra, P.; Mondello, F.; Girolamo, A.; Scafetti, S.; Pistella, E.; Venditti, M. Outbreak of *Saccharomyces cerevisiae* subtype *boulardii* fungemia in patients neighboring those treated with a probiotic preparation of the organism. *J. Clin. Microbiol.* **2003**, *41*, 5340–5343. [CrossRef]
24. Zerva, L.; Hollis, R.J.; Pfaller, M.A. In vitro susceptibility testing and DNA typing of *Saccharomyces cerevisiae* clinical isolates. *J. Clin. Microbiol.* **1996**, *34*, 3031–3034. [CrossRef] [PubMed]
25. Hennequin, C.; Kauffmann-Lacroix, C.; Jobert, A.; Viard, J.P.; Ricour, C.; Jacquemin, J.L.; Berche, P. Possible role of catheters in *Saccharomyces boulardii* fungemia. *Eur. J. Clin. Microbiol. Infect. Dis.* **2000**, *19*, 16–20. [CrossRef] [PubMed]
26. McCullough, M.J.; Clemons, K.V.; McCusker, J.H.; Stevens, D.A. Species identification and virulence attributes of *Saccharomyces boulardii* (nom. inval.). *J. Clin. Microbiol.* **1998**, *36*, 2613–2617. [CrossRef] [PubMed]

27. Mallie, M.; Nguyen, V.-P.; Bertout, S.; Vaillant, C.; Bastide, J.-M. Genotyping study of *Saccharomyces boulardii* compared to the *Saccharomyces sensu stricto* complex species. *J. Mycol. Med.* **2001**, *11*, 19–25.
28. Munoz, P.; Bouza, E.; Cuenca-Estrella, M.; Eiros, J.M.; Pérez, M.J.; Sánchez-Somolinos, M.; Rincón, C.; Hortal, J.; Peláez, T. *Saccharomyces cerevisiae* Fungemia: An Emerging Infectious Disease. *Clin. Infect. Dis.* **2005**, *40*, 1625–1634. [CrossRef]
29. Prattes, J.; Raggam, R.B.; Vanstraelen, K.; Rabensteiner, J.; Hoegenauer, C.; Krause, R.; Prüller, F.; Wölfler, A.; Spriet, I.; Hoenigl, M. Chemotherapy-Induced Intestinal Mucosal Barrier Damage: A Cause of Falsely Elevated Serum 1, 3-Beta-D-Glucan Levels? *J. Clin. Microbiol.* **2016**, *54*, 798–801. [CrossRef]
30. Leelahavanichkul, A.; Worasilchai, N.; Wannalerdsakun, S.; Jutivorakool, K.; Somparn, P.; Issara-Amphorn, J.; Tachaboon, S.; Srisawat, N.; Finkelman, M.; Chindamporn, A. Gastrointestinal Leakage Detected by Serum (1→3)-β-D-Glucan in Mouse Models and a Pilot Study in Patients with Sepsis. *Shock* **2016**, *46*, 506–518. [CrossRef]
31. Piarroux, R.; Millon, L.; Bardonnet, K.; Vagner, O.; Koenig, H. Are live *Saccharomyces* yeasts harmful to patients? *Lancet* **1999**, *353*, 1851–1852. [CrossRef]

MDPI
St. Alban-Anlage 66
4052 Basel
Switzerland
Tel. +41 61 683 77 34
Fax +41 61 302 89 18
www.mdpi.com

Journal of Fungi Editorial Office
E-mail: jof@mdpi.com
www.mdpi.com/journal/jof

www.ingramcontent.com/pod-product-compliance
Lightning Source LLC
LaVergne TN
LVHW070543100526
838202LV00012B/363
* 9 7 8 3 0 3 6 5 0 5 5 4 1 *